D1246605

POWER TRAINING FOR SPORT
Plyometrics For Maximum
Power Development

WITHDRAWN

POWER TRAINING FOR SPORT
Plyometrics For Maximum Power Development

by

TUDOR O. BOMPA, Ph.D.
YORK UNIVERSITY
TORONTO, ONTARIO
CANADA

Illustrations by
Gineta Stoenescu

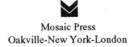

Mosaic Press
Oakville-New York-London

Coaching
Association
of Canada

CANADIAN CATALOGUING IN PUBLICATION DATA

Bompa, Tudor O., 1932-
    Power training for sport: plyometrics for maximum power development

Includes bibliographical references and index.
ISBN 0-88962-629-4

1. Physical education and training.   2. Exercise.
I. Coaching Association of Canada   II. Title.

GV11.5.B65 1993   613.7'11   C93-090023-5

Copyright © 1993 Coaching Asssociation of Canada. Co-published by the
Coaching Association of Canada, 1600 James Naismith Drive, Gloucester,
Ontario K1B 5N4 and Mosaic Press, P.O. Box 1032, Oakville, Ontario L6J
5E9.

New Revised Edition, 1996 © Coaching Association of Canada

All rights Reserved. No part of this publication may be reproduced, stored in
any retrieval system or transmitted in any form or by any means, electronic or
otherwise, without the written permission of the Coaching Association of
Canada, 1600 James Naismith Drive, Gloucester, Ontario K1B 5N4.

Photographs	Courtesy of:	Photographers:
Misty Thomas	Canadian Sport Images	F. Scott Grant
Glenroy Gilbert	Canadian Sport Images	Ted Grant
Melinda Kunhegyi	Canadian Sport Images	Tim O'Lett

Printed in Canada.

In Canada:
MOSAIC PRESS, 1252 Speers Road, Units #1&2, Oakville, Ontario, L6L 5N9,
Canada. P.O. Box 1032, Oakville, Ontario, L6J 5E9
In the United States:
MOSAIC PRESS, 85 River Rock Drive, Suite 202, Buffalo, N.Y., 14207
In the UK and Western Europe:
DRAKE INTERNATIONAL SERVICES, Market House, Market Place,
Deddington, Oxford. OX15 OSF

DEDICATION

To Tamara,

for her many years of support
for my professional endeavours.

TOB

ACKNOWLEDGMENTS

Fig.8, p.20 & Fig.9, p.21
From Edward L. Fox, Richard W. Bowers, and Merle L. Foss,
The Physiological Basis of Physical Education and Athletics, 4th ed.
Copyright 1971, 1976, 1981, and 1988 by W.B. Saunders Company.
Reprinted by permission of Wm. C. Brown Publishers, Dubuque, Iowa.
All Rights Reserved.

Fig.10,p.22
From W.E. Prentice, *Rehabilitation Techniques in Sports Medicine*,
Copyright 1990 by Time Mirror/Mosby College Publishing.
Reprinted by permission of Mosby-Year Book, Inc. St. Louis MO.
All Rights Reserved.

ABOUT THE AUTHOR

Dr. Tudor Bompa is a professor at York University, Toronto, Ontario, Canada. He is a specialist in the theory of training and coaching, to which he has contributed several new concepts, especially in the areas of planning, peaking, and training methodology.

A former professor in his native Romania, he was also a consultant in training/planning to several national coaches and federations. In Romania, he holds the title of Master of Sports, and has coached several medalists in Olympic, World, European and Pan-American championships.

Professor Bompa has been an invited speaker, adviser, and consultant to several countries, including the United States, Australia, Japan, West Germany, Spain, Canada and Belgium. His most recent book, *Theory and Methodology of Training* (Dubuque, Iowa: Kendall/Hunt Publishing Co. 1990) is regarded as the best work in this field.

TABLE OF CONTENTS

INTRODUCTION

An athlete is a trained individual who excels in a particular form of physical activity following a period of extensive physical and psychological training. Training is usually defined as a systematic process of repetitive, progressive exercise which also involves the learning processes and has the ultimate goal of improving the athlete's systems and functions in order to optimize athletic performance.

The key to improvement in athletic performance is a well-organized system of training. A training program must follow the concept of periodization, be well-planned and structured, and be sport specific, so as to cause the athlete's energy systems to adapt to the particular requirements of the sport. For further information on these topics, the reader is advised to read *Theory and Methodology of Training* (Bompa, 1990).

Since ancient times athletes have explored a multitude of methods designed to enable them to run faster, jump higher, and throw an object as far as possible. In order to achieve such goals, power is essential. Explosive, reactive power, is the ability to apply force at a rapid rate, in order to give the body (or object) a high momentum (Power = force x velocity).

An athlete can be very strong and still not be very powerful, simply because of a low rate of utilization, i.e. the ability to contract already strong muscles in a very short period of time. Gains in strength can only be transformed into power by applying specific power training methods. It is probable that one of the most successful of these methods is training employing plyometric exercises.

Also known as reactive training, the stretching-shortening cycle, or myotatic stretch reflex, the exercises known popularly as plyometrics are those in which the muscle is loaded in an eccentric (lengthening) contraction, immediately followed by a concentric (shortening) contraction. In physiological terms, it has been demonstrated that a muscle that is stretched before a contraction will contract more forcefully and rapidly (Bosco and Komi, 1980; Schmidtbleicher, 1984). For example, by lowering the centre of gravity to perform the take-off (in any sports activity) or swinging the golf club before the ball is hit, the athlete stretches the muscle which results in a more forceful contraction.

1

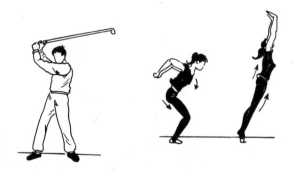

Figure 1. A stretching action before contraction will result in a more explosive contraction.

The term plyometric is a combined one, probably derived from the Greek terms "pleion", meaning more, and "metric", to measure. Thus, it means to measure more or to actually improve more. Although the term has only been in use since the mid-1960s or 1970s, plyometric exercises have existed for a long time. However, some authors, in their attempts to prove just how effective these exercises are, go so far as to claim that plyometrics were invented by the Russians! This is certainly a disservice to all the children in the world who have played "jump rope" or "hop scotch", games which are nothing other than... plyometrics.

The pioneers of plyometrics were probably track and field athletes in the 1920s and '30s, who utilized "jump training" as part of their gym training during the long winters in Eastern and Northern Europe. In 1933, the Romanian National Academy of Physical Education published a booklet on "Jump Training for Athletics". Whether they knew it or not, gymnasts performing tumbling or vaulting have been performing plyometric exercises all along! And that is since the late 1700s! Even further back in history, in the Middle Ages, stone throwers in Switzerland tested their power in informal competitions: in 1470 in the German town of Augsburg, the long jump was won by Prince Christoph of Bavaria! Finally, in the early Middle Ages the fictional figure of Teutobod surpassed everyone in...plyometrics. He jumped over five horses! (Figure 2)

Although plyometric exercises are not new, their athletic benefit has only been studied in the past three decades. Some of the earliest studies were done by Verkhoshanski (1967; 1968) who experimented with the use of various types of plyometrics on an athlete's increments of explosive power. He has claimed improvements in the whole neuro-muscular system, especially in the speed of contraction. During the 1970s and '80s many researchers, especially in Finland, Italy, USA and Germany demonstrated the physiological benefits of reactive training (Cavagna, 1970; Komi and Buskirk, 1972; Bosco et al., 1976; Blattner and Noble, 1979; Bosco et al., 1981, 1982; Schmidtbleicher and Gollhofer, 1982; Clutch et al., 1983; Schmidtbleicher, 1984; Gollhofer et al., 1987 etc.). Other authors addressed this fascinating area, both in articles or books (Wilt, 1978; Chu, 1983, 1984; Radcliffe and Farentinos, 1985; etc.).

As researchers begin to shed more light on the benefits of power training, some ascribe to plyometrics magical qualities and predict miraculous results, while still others dismiss their utility, citing their potential for causing traumatic injuries, mostly due to the ballistic nature of the exercises. So it is legitimate to question what are the essential characteristics of plyometrics.

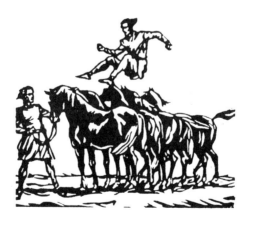

Figure 2.   Teutobod jumping over five horses.

Although there is no magic in plyometrics, it is safe to say from the outset that it is an important form of training which results in the development of explosive power and quicker reactions, based on the improved reactivity of the Central Nervous System (CNS), and the strength to absorb the shock of a balanced landing from a jump (as in figure skating and in many team sports).

For too many years, the importance of the stretching-shortening cycle, a major performance factor in many sports, has been under-estimated. Basic strength training was considered sufficient to develop this explosive element of many athletic movements. Plyometric exercises do address this particular need, which is lacking from traditional strength training programs. By following a training regimen of specific exercises which emphasize explosive-reactive power, the potential of the stretching-shortening cycle can be increased. Plyometric exercises are applicable to sports which involve an eccentric contraction, followed by a concentric contraction. Athletes whose sports involve explosive-reactive types of activity, or a high-end velocity of their own body mass, can benefit from plyometric training (basketball, volleyball, high jumping, football, sprinting, figure skating, ski jumping, etc.). Similarly, athletes in sports involving explosive-reactive types of activity of high-end velocity of some implement or object, such as baseball, hockey, golf and throwing events, also benefit from plyometric exercises.

As much as plyometric exercises are fun and can assist the coach to improve variety in training, they do require a good background in weight training. The chapter on "Methodological Guidelines for Power Training" will further clarify this subject.

POWER TRAINING DEFINED

Maximum contraction, reaction time, and the ability to exert powerful movements at the highest frequency and in the shortest period of time are all dominant abilities for athletes in many sports, and as such are primary factors in enabling athletes to achieve high-level performance.

In the past few years plyometric training has been added to traditional power training methods. However, for reasons of ignorance and lack of scientific evidence, this method is often employed inappropriately. This can result in physiological inefficiency, frequently accompanied by injury. Power training schedules are often planned at the same level, with a similar load and number of repetitions throughout the year, thereby disregarding the need to constantly increase the intensity of stimuli (load), and the specific needs of periodization (scheduling different types of strength and power training during the training phases of the annual plan).

Power is produced in a stretching-shortening type of contraction where the extensor muscle shows greater stiffness and enlarges the tension at the tendon. This results in a more economical and effective eccentric phase. Moreover, during the stretching of a muscle, reflex activities provide for a higher activation than is possible during voluntary contractions. This again enhances the tension at the tendon and together with the neuronal input during the concentric phase, a forceful push-off can be produced.

Power performance in the stretching-shortening cycle is a relatively independent motor quality (Schmidtbleicher and Gollhofer, 1982; Clutch et al., 1983; Gollhofer et al., 1987), which involves the nervous system to levels beyond those generated by most other types of exercise. The adaptation of the nervous system to the training stimulus, (an overlooked scientific fact in most training programs) plays a significant role, since the system reacts very sensitively in terms of adaptation to a slow or fast contractile stimulus. High intensity training, like power exercises, results in the quick mobilization of greater innervation activities, the recruitment of most of the motor units and their corresponding muscle fibres, and in an increase in the firing rate of the motor neurons (Schmidtbleicher, 1984; Gollhofer et al., 1987). This increased innervation produces considerable improvement in the development of power.

From the practical point of view, two reflexes are of particular interest:

1) the myotatic reflex, a typical stretch reflex and the one physicians use when they tap the knee (patella) tendon. This reflex is very rate-sensitive, which means that if the stretch is performed slowly the response will be very insignificant, or non-existent. On the other hand, a quick jerk results in a fast and powerful contraction.

2) the reflex of the Golgi tendon organ, a receptor located in the muscle tendon, which acts as an inverse myotatic reflex. When a muscle is stretched beyond a certain degree of flexibility, this reflex brings about relaxation of the muscle, not contraction, thereby avoiding injury.

The use of plyometric exercises seems to develop the "reactive neuro-muscular apparatus" (Verkhoshanski and Tatyan, 1983) or the concentric and eccentric activity which loads the elastic and contractile components of muscle (Atha, 1981). The elastic nature of muscle fibre allows a muscle to store potential energy during the eccentric phase of a movement, which is then released as kinetic (relating to the motion) energy in the ensuing concentric contraction, causing a rapid, explosive movement.

To ensure that full advantage of the stretch reflex is attained, the muscle must be forcibly stretched: it is important to emphasize the velocity of stretch, which brings about a rapid rise in the firing frequency of the muscle spindle (Astrand and Rodahl, 1970, O'Connell and Gardner, 1972). This effect can be achieved and exploited through various forms of plyometrics, especially depth jumps employing plyo-boxes (Bompa, 1988). Several authors suggest that depth jumps result in statistically significant increases in vertical jumps, representing nothing other than power increments (Verkhoshanski, 1969; Blattner and Noble, 1979).

But why use plyometrics anyway? This present chapter gives a partial, condensed explanation of the physiological justification for plyometrics. The following chapter describes in detail the physiological basis of plyometric training. However, the main reason for employing plyometric exercises is the need to activate the motor units more quickly, in order to cause a better neurological adaptation.

In analyzing some athletic movements (Figure 3), it is evident that the duration of the contact phase in the speed-power exercises is extremely short. In comparison, the limb extension typical of weight training, is much slower. If the extension is performed against heavy resistance, the duration is prolonged even more!

No.	Event		Duration/ms
1	100m dash		100 - 200
2	Long jump		150 - 180
3	High jump:	-flop	150 - 180
4		-straddle	220
5	Vaulting in gymnastics		100 - 120
6	Leg extension		600
7	Arm extension		450

Figure 3.   The duration of the contact phase (milliseconds) of some track events and the contraction time of limb extension (from Schmidtbleicher, 1984).

Therefore, the discrepancy between the duration of the contact phase and limb extension, begs the question whether the supposedly positive transfer from weight training to speed-power exercises lives up to expectations. Plyometric exercises, however, do employ movements which are extremely short and explosive, where the activation of the neuro-muscular units are much higher than in the normal voluntary contraction.

Any attempt to answer the question "why plyometrics?" could also explore the force-time curves of different types of jumps (Figure 4).

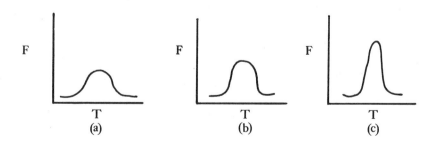

Figure 4.   The force-time curves of three types of jumps: (a) = squat jump; (b) = stretching-shortening cycle; (c) = reactive jump (from Schmidtbleicher, 1984).

7

Both the duration as well as the magnitude of the curves demonstrate that a jump typical of the stretching-shortening cycle and the plyometric jump are performed much faster, with a superior peak force, as compared to the squat jump.

A comparison of the force-time curves of two kinds of strength training demonstrates that training employing a higher number of repetitions (12-15) performed to exhaustion is the least useful when compared to loads using maximum force/reactive jumps of few repetitions (Figure 5).

Since in most sports the time of force application is short (120-150 ms), only the phase showed by the left arrow (Figure 5) is effective and has application to sports. The type of force developed through higher numbers of repetitions (right arrow) is of little use since it is applied at a much lower speed.

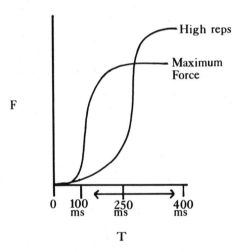

Figure 5.   The force-time curve of two different weight training programs (from Schmidtbleicher, 1984).

ANATOMICAL AND MECHANICAL PROPERTIES OF PLYOMETRIC TRAINING

The musculo-skeletal frame of the body is an arrangement of bones attached to one another by a series of ligaments at structures called joints (which allow the motion of articulating bones), and a number of muscles crossing the joints, which provide the force necessary for the body's movements.

From the point of view of plyometric exercise, the spinal column represents a mechanism which gives the body stability, support for the weight of the body, and more importantly, acts as a shock absorber for cushioning all the "hops" and "jumps".

This amazing mechanism is the core of many effective functions. Close to its base is also the body's centre of gravity. While performing a great variety of plyometric exercises, the path of the centre of gravity can be altered only as long as the body is in contact with the ground. As soon as the body is projected into the air, as a result of a hop or leap, the path of the centre of gravity is determined by the magnitude of the force exerted at the time of take-off against the resistance of the ground. Once the body is projected into the air, the path of the centre of gravity cannot be altered, regardless of the eventual movements performed by the limbs.

As the force of the legs projects the body into the air, this force has to overcome the inertia of the body and the pull of gravity. Since this force is dependent upon the weight of the body, only strength and power training increase the force required to overcome the gravitational pull, and as a result allow the athlete to jump higher. This force is produced by the quick contraction in the extension of the legs and a forceful upward arm swing. The quicker the leg extension, the greater the force that can be produced against the ground. Prior to that, in preparation for generating this force, the hips, knee, and the ankle must be flexed (bent), and then followed by a powerful leg extension (force exertion).

The depth of the crouch performed at the instant of joint flexion depends on the power of the legs. The deeper the crouch, the greater the force required from the leg extensors. However, the crouch represents a mechanical necessity, because it puts the muscles in a state of stretch, giving them a greater distance to accelerate, culminating in a take-off.

To be more effective, the depth of the crouch must be proportional to the power of the legs. If the flexion is too great, the extension (or shortening phase) will be performed slowly, and as a result the jump will be low.

The technique and exertion of force while jumping is essential for performing strictly linear and well-balanced plyometric exercise. For a take-off from both feet, the push against the ground has to be simultaneously and equally exerted so that both sides of the body have a linear motion. In a single foot take-off, on the other hand, the centre of gravity is brought in line with the take-off foot by driving the opposite knee forward and swinging forward the arm from the same side as the take-off leg. This arm action will compensate for the knee drive, and as a result avoid any rotary movement induced by the take-off leg.

The forceful forward knee drive also produces an upward momentum and together with the arm swing will add force to the jump. However, the arm is swung dynamically forward for plyometric exercises performed in a horizontal plane, and upward when height is the objective.

The action involved in a plyometric type of exercise relies mechanically on the stretch reflex which is found in the belly of the individual muscle. The main purpose of the stretch reflex is to monitor the degree of muscle stretch and to thereby prevent overstretching of any muscle fibres which could otherwise be torn. When an athlete jumps off the ground, a large amount of force is required to propel the entire body mass off the ground. The body must be able to flex and extend the body limbs very quickly, in order to leave the ground. A plyometric type of exercise relies on this quick body action, in order to attain the power which is required for the movement.

Mechanically, when the take-off leg is planted, the athlete must lower the centre of gravity, which creates a downward velocity. This "amortization phase" is an important component of any jumping type of activity, for it is during this phase that the athlete prepares for take-off in a different direction. A long amortization phase, (also called the "shock absorbing phase"), is responsible for a loss of power. An example of this lower power output is seen in the long jumper who does not plant the take-off leg properly. This mistake by the jumper will result in a loss of both the upward and the horizontal velocity which is required to propel the jumper forward. An athlete who performs a jumping action must work towards a shorter and quicker amortization phase: the shorter this phase, the more powerful the concentric muscle contraction, when the muscle has previously been stretched during the eccentric contraction or the amortization phase. (Bosco and Komi, 1980). This action is possible due to the recovery and utilization of all the energy which has been stored in the elastic components of the muscle during any stretching action.

All jumping motion can be improved through the analysis of each individual, biomechanical component of the jump. An example of this is the improvement in a high jumper's technique: enhanced performance of a high jump can be achieved through the elimination of the deep knee bend phase of the jump, and the shortening of the time interval between the eccentric and the concentric contractions. The elimination of the deep flexion utilizes the elastic qualities of the muscle more efficiently.

As mentioned earlier, all jumpers need first to lower their centre of gravity, thereby creating a downward velocity. The athlete must then produce forces which will counter the downward motion (amortization phase), in order to get prepared for the upward, thrusting phase. To look at the jump from a mechanical point of view, it must be remembered that **force equals mass times acceleration** ($F = m \times a$). A greater force is required in order to decelerate the body more quickly and therefore will result in a shorter amortization phase. From this a second equation can be created: (Young and Marino, 1989)

$$\text{Average force of amortization} = \frac{\text{body mass x change in velocity}}{\text{time of amortization}}$$

If the athlete wants to decrease the time of amortization, a greater average force is required. If the athlete is not able to generate this force, a longer, less efficient amortization phase will occur which will result in a loss of horizontal velocity, due to the weakened concentric contraction.

This amortization equation also points out the importance of maintaining a low level of body fat and a high power-weight ratio, for even greater average force of amortization would be required if the body mass of the athlete is increased. A greater downward velocity at impact requires an increase in the average force produced during the amortization phase. An example of this is seen in long or high jumpers who lower their centre of gravity prior to take-off, thereby reducing the impact of the forces. (Young and Marino, 1985)

The entire body of the athlete must be used efficiently in order to maximize jumping ability. The upward acceleration of the free limbs, for example the arms, after the amortization phase acts to increase the vertical forces placed on the take-off leg. A triple jumper for example must be able to apply peak force as great as 50 times body weight in order to compensate for the inability to lower the centre of gravity during a hop, as compared to a long jumper who can manipulate his body more easily just prior to take-off. An effective take-off will only be achieved if the jumper can apply large forces on impact and produce a shorter, quicker amortization phase.

It is sometimes difficult to train for this specific phase of the jump, as few conventional exercises are applicable. Many jumpers use traditional weight training (e.g. squats or any Olympic lifts) in order to train for this take-off phase of their jumps. This type of weight training places a large load on the leg extensors which will over time provide an adequate strength training base. The main problem with only using weight training is that it is unlikely that a heavy squat lift would be fast enough to utilize the elastic qualities of the muscles. Such a lift is also restricted to a single joint movement. This is not the case in the single leg take-off, which involves multiple joint movements all happening simultaneously.

Bounding exercises, on the other hand, can be used successfully to simulate an effective take-off and can therefore improve the overall jumping ability of the athlete. Bounding has the potential to possess very similar force-time characteristics to the take-off leg and to exert force in a short time interval. The bounding exercises will also involve multi-joint movement and provide the possibility of the development of the required muscle elasticity. (Young and Marino, 1985)

As in any activity that involves repetitive, ballistic movements, there is a certain risk of injury, especially if appropriate methodological advice (such as is suggested later in the text) is ignored. Injuries occur primarily when outside forces acting upon a joint momentarily exceed the structural integrity of the muscles, bones and connective tissues. When performing plyometric exercises, numerous parts of the musculo-skeletal system are exposed to extreme biomechanical loading. The connective tissues of the foot, ankle, hip and the intervertebral discs all act as natural shock absorbers in an attempt to dissipate the imposed stress.

Young athletes are even more prone to trauma since their musculo-skeletal systems are relatively immature. The epiphyseal plates of their long bones have not yet fused, thereby making the head and neck of the femur especially vulnerable to injury. Other potential injuries may include patellar tendinitis, shin splints, heel bruises as well as various strains. Some of the eventual injuries acquired from overuse can be limited or avoided by respecting a thorough progression and periodization (refer to Chapter 7, "Planning").

ENERGY SYSTEMS AND PLYOMETRIC PHYSIOLOGY

The human body performs exercise through the use of three major energy systems. The first system is the anaerobic alactic energy system, which comes into play during the first ten seconds of exercise. This alactic phase relies on the adenosine triphosphate (ATP) and the creatine phosphate (CP) pools stored in the muscle cells as a quick energy source. The breakdown of ATP provides energy which can be used in exercise. ATP is then reformed with the energy released from the breakdown of CP. This system, which provides energy for short and explosive activities, is very restricted, for once the CP stores are exhausted, the body must look elsewhere for its energy needs.

Energy Pathway	Anaerobic Pathway		Aerobic Pathway		
	Alactic	Lactic			
Primary Energy Source	ATP Produced Without the Presence of O_2		ATP Produced in the Presence of O_2		
Fuel	Phosphate System. ATP/CP Stored in Muscle	Lactic Acid (LA) System Glycogen — LA Byproduct	Glycogen Completely Burned in the Presence of O_2	Fats	Protein
Duration	0 Sec 10 Sec.	40 Sec. 70 Sec.	2 Min. 6 Min.	1h 2h 3h	
Sports/ Events	- Sprinting 100 Dash - Throws - Jumps - Weight Lifting - Ski Jumping - Diving - Vaulting in Gym-nastics	- 200-400M - 500 Speed Skating - Most Gym Events - Cycling Track	- 100 M Swimming - 800 M Track - 500 Canoeing - 1000 Speed Skating - Floor Ex. Gym. - Alpine Skiing - Cycling Track: 1000M and Pursuit	- Middle Dist. Track. Swimming Speed Skat. - 1000 Canoeing - Boxing - Wrestling - Marshal Arts - Figure Skating - Synch. Swim - Cycling-Pursuit	- Long Distance: Track Swimming Speed Skating. Canoeing - Cross Country Skiing - Rowing - Cycling, Road Racing	
	Most Team Sports/Racquet Sports/Sailing				

Figure 6.   Energy sources for competitive sports.

The second energy system used by the body is the anaerobic lactic system, which is utilized principally within the first two minutes of exercise, and relies on the carbohydrate stores for its energy. Carbohydrates area stored as glycogen in the muscle, and glucose in the bloodstream, being the only food fuel available for the anaerobic lactic system. The end product of this system is a by-product called lactic acid. When high intensity work is continued for a prolonged period of time, large quantities of lactic acid accumulate and limit the duration of exercise by restricting each muscle's output, thereby resulting in fatigue. All plyometric exercises utilize the energy provided by the anaerobic alactic and anaerobic lactic systems, the former being the dominant of the two.

The third energy system is the aerobic, which relies on the carbohydrate and fat stores in the body. This energy system comes into play after approximately two minutes of exercise. This aerobic, or endurance phase, utilized both carbohydrates and the fat stores, for in the oxidation of free fatty acids or lipids, the power output is less than thatfrom the oxidation of carbohydrate. The total free fatty acid stores are therefore more plentiful, thus these fats become a predominant energy source in any exercise of long duration and lower power output.

Exercise Forms

In order to train these energy systems, specific forms of exercise have been developed. Strength training is the capacity to exert force of the ability to do work against resistance. In order to increase a muscle's capacity to do work, the muscle must be overloaded. Muscle hypertrophy is an increase in the muscle size and cross-sectional area, which has been caused by a development of the existing constituent fibres through the use of strength training exercises. The muscle size also increases when a greater total number of capillaries is called into play.

Speed training is also a form of exercise which trains the anaerobic alactic energy system. The expenditure of an enormous amount of energy in a short period of time results in speed training. Speed training relies almost exclusively on the oxygen within the tissues. Any anaerobic alactic activity therefore depends on the immediate chemical release of any oxidative energy phosphate compound which is an instant energy source for the working muscles). Speed training, like any other form of training, is dependent on the resilience and responsiveness of the circulatory system.

Endurance training is the development of the aerobic energy system. The term aerobic describes any activity that is performed in the presence of oxygen. Aerobic capacity is the limiting factor in how well an individual athlete will perform over a long period of time. Endurance training puts stress on the heart muscle which thereby becomes stronger and is able to pump more blood--hence oxygen--at a faster rate. There is also an increase in the number of capillaries supplying the muscle tissue due to this increase in stress on the heart. The positive effect of any aerobic training is the increased efficiency of the body: the oxygen is transported faster, the waste products are eliminated quicker, and the overall circulatory system improves as a result of training.

In most sports, the energy requirements can only be met through the use of two of the energy systems, or through some contribution from all three energy systems. The shorter the performance time, the greater the power output can be and the more rapid the energy requirement. Conversely, the longer the duration, the smaller the power output and the lower the rate of energy requirement. In a short-term, high-intensity activity, the energy is supplied through the anaerobic alactic system. Longer duration, low-intensity activity relies entirely on the aerobic energy system.

The lactic energy system is used only in conjunction with another energy system. In prolonged activities where the lactic system could be brought into play, i.e. in order to avoid fatigue, the energy contribution from the lactic system must be kept low, at least until near the end of the performance. In summary, therefore, in any activity of thirty to seventy seconds in length the predominant energy systems are the anaerobic alactic and lactic systems. In activities of seventy seconds to three minutes, the predominant energy systems are the anaerobic lactic and the aerobic systems. Finally in any activity which lasts longer than three minutes the predominant energy system is the aerobic energy system.

Muscle Physiology

In order to explain plyometrics better, it is important to understand muscle physiology. The human body is constructed around a bony skeleton. The skeleton frame is covered with approximately six hundred muscles which represent about forty percent of the body's weight. A muscle is a collection of long fibres which are made up of cells and grouped in bundles. Each bundle is separately wrapped in a sheath that holds it together and protects it. All of the muscles of our body are a mixture of two distinctly different fibres: fast-twitch for the anaerobic energy systems and slow-twitch (slow oxidative, or SO) for the longer duration aerobic energy system.

Fast-twitch muscle fibre can be further defined as either fast oxidative glycolytic (FOG or type IIa) or fast glycolytic (FG or type IIb). The fast-twitch fibre can produce high speed movement for a short period of time.

Slow-twitch muscle fibre produces less power and therefore less speed, but can perform for a longer period of time. The slow-twitch fibre is highly oxidative and is therefore employed in any aerobic energy requirement.

A muscular contraction is shortening of the muscle fibres. There are three distinctly different forms of contraction available to the working muscle. An isometric contraction is a contraction completed in a static position, and therefore results in no change in the length of the muscles or the angle of the joint at which the contraction takes place. An isometric form of contraction is very specific to the joint angle at which the contraction takes place. An isotonic contraction is either a shortening or lengthening of the muscle fibres through the entire range of motion. An isotonic contraction never involves the exact same muscle fibres throughout the entire movement. The load remains constant, regardless of the angle of contraction, or the degree of fatigue. An isokinetic contraction refers to constant velocity over the full range of motion. The resistance varies, however, according to the angle of pull and the degree of fatigue.

Other terms which must be explained are eccentric and concentric. An eccentric muscle movement is one in which the muscle develops tension while lengthening (sometimes also called ''negative'' work). A concentric muscle movement is one in which the muscle develops tension while shortening (also known as ''positive'' work).

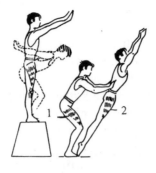

1 eccentric   2 concentric

Figure 7.   An illustration of the eccentric and concentric contraction.

Neuro-Muscular Physiology

The area of neuro-muscular physiology and motor control is rarely treated in discussions of sporting activity. Neuro-muscular physiology is the area responsible for the neural stimulus which provides kinematic movement patterns, muscle enzymatic profiles and muscle fibre type composition.

In terms of exercise training, sport specificity is still the primary rule to remember. An example of exercise specificity can be seen in the use of high resistance exercises which result in an increase in maximal strength, but only moderate improvements in the maximal rate of force production. On the other hand, an exercise program that is geared towards improving explosive strength improves the rate of force production, with only a limited increase in maximal strength.

When dealing specifically with the neural influence of the body, it should be pointed out that the neuro-muscular system does not always behave as predicted. The muscular force-velocity relationship, for example, has always been recognized as an inverse one: as the resistance increases, so does the force, but the velocity decreases.

Once this relationship is applied to a human muscle, the results differ significantly. One explanation for this change in results may be due to the force-sensitive proprioceptors (Golgi tendon organs) which prevent the production of an injury-causing level of force. The classic stretch reflex may be altered in some athletes due to the specificity involved in each individual sport.

The role of a reflex pathway in terms of motor control can be demonstrated in a variety of ways. A muscle which is forcibly stretched during an active contraction, produces a greater force than would be developed during an isometric or static contraction. A lengthening or eccentric contraction produces a greater force than an isometric contraction. The neural component of this action can be demonstrated in a knee extension contraction. When the right leg is stretched while the individual maintains a maximal effort in both legs, the strength of the left leg extensors obviously declines.

The neural mechanism explained here is an example of classic Sheringtonian neurophysiology known as the crossed extensor reflex: contracting one muscle group inhibits the contralateral homonymous musculature. This reflex helps us to maintain an upright posture by increasing the extensor force in the quadriceps when balance in the contralateral leg has suddenly been disrupted. A second example which stays consistent with the idea that a neural reflex pathway is important in strength production, comes from the observation of bilateral contractions. A simultaneous bilateral contraction produces less force than the sum of the individual unilateral contractions.

Over the years, the role of the nervous system in strength training has generally been overlooked. The greatest strength gains occur in the early stages of a strength training program. During this period researchers have noted little change in the muscle fibre size or type, the anaerobic enzyme activity or the energy substrate levels. At a time when strength is increasing, there seems to be little change in muscle physiology. Research now shows that during this early strength training interval, there are changes in coordination patterns involving agonist and antagonist muscles and as a result they seem to learn to increase the pattern of activity of the motor units responsible for the contraction. The early part of the training period therefore seems to be mediated by neural mechanisms, while muscle hypertrophy plays a greater role later on in training.

Plyometric Physiology

Plyometric movement is based on the reflex contraction of the muscle fibres resulting from the rapid loading (and thus stretching) of these same muscle fibres. Physiologically, when excessive stretching and tearing become a possibility, the stretch receptors cause proprioceptive nerve impulses to be sent to the spinal cord and then through a rebounding action they are received back at the stretch

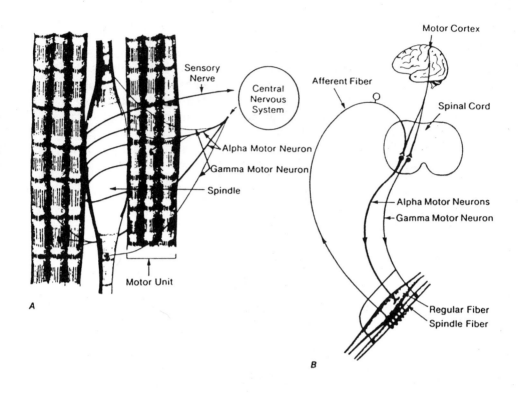

Figure 8.   A. Structure of the muscle spindle; B. Connections to the
central nervous system of the muscle spindle. The spindle
is sensitive to stretching. It can be stretched when the
entire muscle is stretched or when the gamma motor
neurons are stimulated by the motor cortex (gamma loop).
In either case, sensory impulses from the spindle are sent
to the spinal cord, stimulating the alpha motor neurons,
and the muscle contracts. Also, direct stimulation of the
alpha motor neurons from the motor cortex is possible
(From Fox, E.L., R.W. Bowers and M.L. Foss.   The
Physiological Basis of Physical Education and Athletics.
Wm.C. Brown Publishers, 1988).

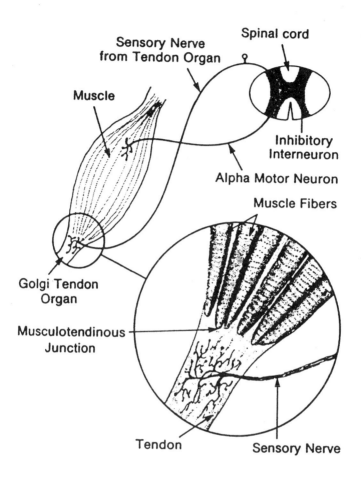

Figure 9. The Golgi tendon organ. When a contracted muscle is
forcibly stretched, the sensory nerve of the tendon organ is
stimulated. Impulses are sent to the spinal cord, where a
synapse is made with an inhibitory interneuron that inhibits the alpha motor neuron, and the muscle relaxes (From
Fox, E.L., R.W. Bowers and M.L. Foss. The Physiological
Basis of Physical Education and Athletics. Wm.C. Brown
Publishers, 1988).

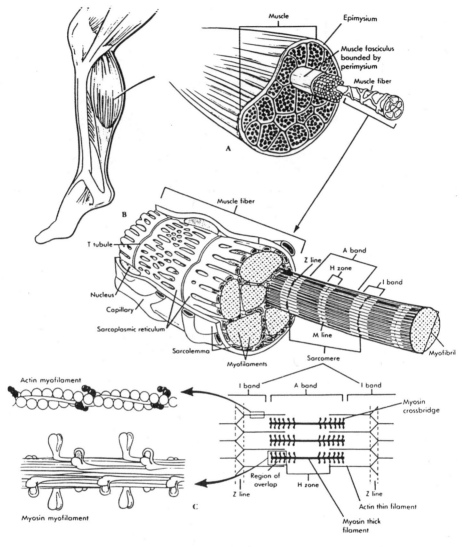

Figure 10. Muscle physiology. A. Muscle is composed of muscle fasciculi, which can be seen by the unaided eye as striations in the muscle. The fasciculi are composed of bundles of individual muscle fibres (muscle cells). B. Each muscle fibre contains myofibrils in which the banding patterns of the sarcomeres are seen. C. The myofibrils are composed of actin myofilaments and myosin myofilaments, which are formed from thousands of individual actin and myosin molecules (From Prentice, W.E., Rehabilitation Techniques in Sports Medicine. *Time Mirror/Mosby College Publishing, 1990).*

receptors. By this rebounding action, a braking effect is applied, further stretching of the muscle fibres is prevented and, most importantly, in terms of plyometrics, a powerful muscle contraction is released.

The primary sensory receptor responsible for detecting rapid elongation of muscle fibres is the muscle spindle (see Figure 8), which is capable of responding to both the magnitude and the rate of change in length of the muscle fibres. The Golgi tendon organ (see Figure 9) is located in the tendons and responds to excessive tension as a result of powerful contractions and the stretching of the muscle. Both of these sensory receptors function at the reflex level, and both transmit large amounts of information to the brain via the spinal cord.

Anatomically, the muscle spindles show how the mechanoreceptors may function during any plyometric movement. Each spindle is comprised of several specifically adapted muscle fibres referred to as intrafusal fibres. These intrafusal fibres lack the ability to contract, containing neither of the contractile proteins actin or myosin. The end portions of the intrafusals which attach to the connective sheaths do contract, as they contain the actin and myosin which facilitate contraction. Some intrafusals have large central bulges filled with cell nuclei, the so-called nuclear bag fibres. The nuclear chain fibres differ in function from the other intrafusal fibres, as they contain single chains of cell nuclei at their centres.

Muscle spindle innervation involves both sensory and motor nerves. The main sensory innervation is located at the centre of the nuclear bag intrafusal fibres. These nerve endings form a coil around the intrafusals and are the actual receptors for detecting changes in the length of the intrafusals. Due to the attachment characteristics of the intrafusal fibres, any change in length of the intrafusals or any movement in the coil-like ending results in a change in length. The primary sensory neuron also sends out branches that wind around the centers of the nuclear chain intrafusals. The sensory neurons which are associated with the primary receptors are capable of transmitting nervous impulses to the spinal cord and thus to the brain.

Two additional sensory endings are also located in the muscle spindle. Sensory endings are located on either side of the annulospiral ending. Both of these sensory endings are associated with the non-contractile portions of the nuclear chain intrafusal. Innervating the contractile ends of both nuclear chain and nuclear bag intrafusal fibres are efferent (motor) neurons from the spinal cord. The motor neurons are part of the gamma-efferent system and are not associated with the alpha motor neurons that innervate the skeletal muscle fibres themselves. It should be noted that the primary as well as the secondary receptors can be activated in different ways. Any lengthening of the skeletal muscle fibres will cause a stretching of the intrafusals and in turn the coiled endings of the primary receptors. The contractile ends of the intrafusals are innervated by the gamma-efferent motor neurons; stimulation of the intrafusals in this manner can cause them to contract, thereby stretching their central portions and in turn activating the primary receptors. This action can occur even though the skeletal muscle fibres remain unstretched.

In terms of overall function, the muscle spindle is capable of emitting two types of responses, static and dynamic. A static response may occur when the intrafusal fibre is slowly stretched, resulting from a gradual stretching of the skeletal muscle fibres or perhaps from direct stimulation of the intrafusals by the gamma-efferent system. As a result of this, the primary and secondary coiled receptors are pulled apart, thus emitting a continuous, low-level stream of nervous impulses. As the magnitude of stretching increases, the rate of emission of nervous impulses also increases. This static response can continue for several minutes, as long as the skeletal muscle fibres remain stretched.

In the dynamic response of the muscle spindle, the primary receptor is activated by a rapid change in length of the intrafusal fibre around which it is coiled. When this occurs, the primary receptor sends many impulses to the spinal cord. The dynamic response is abrupt, for when the stretching occurs the response is immediate. The dynamic response ceases almost as quickly as it was initiated, after which the muscle spindle resumes its static level of discharge. The dynamic response is believed to be important with respect to plyometrics. Due to the involvement of the primary receptors with the nuclear bag intrafusals, the dynamic response is also involved in the detection of rapid stretching of the muscle.

The main function of the muscle spindle is to elicit the so-called stretch or myotatic reflex, which is considered the neuro-muscular process that typifies the action basis of plyometrics. When the muscle fibres are rapidly stretched, the lengthening of the fibres is detected by the muscle spindle, thereby eliciting a dynamic response. A large burst of impulses is sent to the spinal cord via the afferent neurons of the primary receptor. These neurons synapse directly with alpha motor neurons which in turn send back impulses to the skeletal muscle fibres and cause them to contract.

A stretch reflex may also occur as a slower, more static response. If the muscle is stretched gradually, the nuclear chain intrafusals send slower but continuous impulses to the spinal cord, which in turn synapse with the alpha motor neurons. This entire reaction results in a lower-intensity contraction of the skeletal muscle fibre. This slower, static contraction may take several minutes, as opposed to the dynamic contraction which will occur in less than a second.

The influence of the gamma-efferent stimulation on the magnitude and intensity of the dynamic stretch reflex is very important. If, in the example of the depth jump, the level of gamma-efferent static stimulation to the muscle spindles of the quadriceps were very low, then the sensitivity of the spindle to sudden stretching would be depressed and the effectiveness of the dynamic stretch reflex would be almost nil. The gamma-efferent system is also important in dampening or enhancing the degree of responsiveness of the muscle spindles. Some activities must be executed in a smooth and continuous manner, and therefore the gamma-efferent function is to dampen the responsiveness of the muscle spindle to changes in length of the muscles being used. When the activity must be executed quickly, the response is to decrease the amount of dampening and therefore enhance the response of the system.

Plyometrics work within the complex neural mechanisms. As a result of any plyometric training, changes occur at both the muscular and the neural levels that facilitate and enhance the performance of more rapid and powerful movement skills. The Golgi tendon is a mechanoreceptor which is located in the tendon itself and is stimulated by tensile forces generated by the contraction of muscle fibres to which it is attached. The Golgi tendon responds maximally to sudden increases in tension and transmits a lower, more continuous level of impulses when tension is decreased.

The Golgi tendon reflex occurs when muscle tension is increased. Signals transmitted to the spinal cord cause an inhibitory response to the contracted muscle, thus preventing an inordinate amount of tension from developing in the muscle. The Golgi tendon organ is thought to be a protective device, preventing tearing of the muscle and/or tendon under extreme conditions.

The contractile elements of the muscles are the muscle fibres. Certain parts of the muscles are non-contractile, and thus result in what is known as the "series elastic component." The stretching of the series elastic component during muscle contraction produces an elastic potential energy similar to that of a loaded spring. When this energy is released, it augments to some degree the energy of contraction generated by the muscle fibres. This action is seen in plyometric movements. When the muscle is being stretched rapidly, the series elastic component is also stretched, thus storing a portion of the load force in the form of elastic potential energy. The recovery of the stored elastic energy occurs during the concentric or overcoming phase of muscle contraction, which is triggered by the myotatic reflex.

Summary of plyometric training:
* a muscle will contract more forcefully and quickly from a pre-stretched position;
* the more rapid the pre-stretch, the more forceful the concentric contraction;
* it is essential to learn correct technique for doing plyometric exercises;
* it is important to ensure the athlete lands in a pre-stretched, or bent legs (arms) position;
* the shortening contraction should occur immediately after the completion of the pre-stretch phase;
* the transition from the pre-stretch phase should be smooth, continuous and as swift as possible;
* plyometric training results in:
  - the quick mobilization of greater innervation activities;
  - the recruitment of most, if not all, motor units and their corresponding muscle fibres;
  - an increase in firing rate of the motor neurons;
  - the transformation of muscle strength into explosive power;
* plyometrics develop the nervous system so that it will react with maximal speed to the lengthening of muscle; in turn, it will develop the ability to shorten (contract) rapidly and with maximal force;
* repeated reactive training induces fatigue which affects both the eccentric, but more noticeably, the concentric work capacity; fatigue is characterized by increases in the duration of the contact time (Gollhofer et al., 1987).

Training Adaptation
A high level of performance is the result of many years of hard, well-planned and methodical training. During this time the athlete tries to adapt bodily organs and functions to the specific requirements of the chosen sport. The level of adaptation is reflected in the athlete's

performance capabilities. The greater the degree of adaptation, the better the performance capability.

Adaptation to training is the sum of modifications brought about by the systematic repetition of exercise. These structural and physiological changes are the result of a specific demand placed upon the body by the specific activity pursued, and are dependent on the volume, intensity and frequency of training. Physical training is beneficial only as long as it challenges the body to adapt to the stress of a physical demand. If the stress is not sufficient to challenge the body, then no adaptation occurs. If a stress is so great that it cannot be tolerated, injury or over-training may result. Therefore, the "highly-trained athletes have a faster response-time in which to adapt" (Powers et al., 1985).

The time required for a high degree of adaptation depends on the complexity of the skill and the physiological and psychological difficulty of the exercise. The more complex and difficult the activity, the longer the training time required for neuro-muscular and functional adaptation.

Following a systematic and organized program there are several alterations induced by training. Although the greatest number of organic and functional changes have been observed in endurance athletes, almost all athletes are subject to neuro-muscular, cardio-respiratory and biochemical modifications. However, there are also psychological changes which result from a particular physical state, since there seems to be a correlation between physical and psychological development.

Research in the area of anatomical adaptation has shown that there is a decrease in material strength with high intensity exercise, and that the mechanical properties of bones are not strictly dependent on chronological age but rather on the mechanical demands on the athlete. Therefore, low intensity training, at an early age, may stimulate long bone strength and girth increases. High intensity training, on the other hand, may inhibit bone growth (Matsuda, 1986).

Bone adaptation to exercise is also believed to be a function of age. Immature bones are more sensitive to cycle load changes than are more mature bones. For example, long bone growth is suppressed after training and physical training accelerates the maturation process, causing permanent suppression of bone growth (Matsuda, 1986). Therefore, the purpose of training is to stress the body so that the response results in adaptation and not aggravation.

Strength and power training performed at near or maximal voluntary contraction increase the cross-sectional area of muscle fibres (hypertrophy). The growth of a muscle and its weight is largely due to hypertrophy, and the increase of protein content.

Enhancement of explosive power performance and the corresponding biological adaptation of a specific training stimulus are not yet fully understood. Gravity normally provides the major portion of mechanical stimulus response for the development of muscle structure during every day life and during training. Therefore it is reasonable to assume that high gravity conditions (e.g. plyometrics) could influence the muscle mechanics of even well-trained athletes. Improvements as a result of fast adaptation to the stimulated high gravity field were reported. It is suggested that adaptation had occurred both in neuro-muscular functions and in metabolic processes (Bosco et al., 1984).

Performance improvements are also due to changes in the neuro-muscular system. During sustained maximal or sub-maximal activities, the average firing rate of a motor unit increases over time. This neuro-muscular strategy can increase the time over which the contraction is held.

The human organism adapts and improves in direct relationship to the type of stimuli (training) to which it is exposed. The work performed in training is considered to be the cause, while the organism adaptation is the effect. In order to achieve an optimal training effect, training programs must be planned which are specific to the sport and which are prescribed with appropriate intensity. The quantity of work to be performed in a training session must be set in accordance with individual abilities, the phase of training, and a correct ratio between the volume and intensity of training. Therefore, if the training load is properly administered, appropriate athletic development will occur, and lead to an improvement in performance.

The Overcompensation Cycle

The adaptation process is the result of a constant alternation between stimulation and compensation, between work and regeneration. This constant alternation is illustrated by the overcompensation, or supercompensation cycle.

Overcompensation refers mostly to the effects of work and regeneration of the organism as a biological foundation for physical and psychological arousal for the main competition of the year.

All individuals have a specific level of biological functioning that prevails during normal daily activities. An individual involved in training is exposed to a series of stimuli which disturb the normal biological state (homeostasis) by burning supplementary food stuff, the outcome of which is organism and CNS fatigue and high lactic acid concentration in the blood and at the muscle cell level. Therefore, at the end of a training session an athlete experiences a certain level of fatigue which temporarily reduces the organism's capacity to function. The abrupt drop of the homeostasis curve (Figure 11) illustrates the rapid transition into a state of fatigue, which assumes a simultaneous reduction in functional capacity. Following training, and between two training sessions, there is a phase of compensation during which the biochemical sources of energy are replenished. The return of the curve towards a normal biological state is achieved slowly and progressively, suggesting that the organism's replenishment of the loss of energy is a slower process, requiring several hours. However, if the time between two training stimuli (training sessions) of high intensity is longer, the energy sources are not only replaced but may surpass the initial level, facilitating the organism to rebound and thus be in a state of over-compensation. Overcompensation should be considered as the foundation of a functional increase in athletic efficiency as a result of the adaptation of the organism to the training stimulus and the replenishment of the glycogen stores in the muscle. If the resting phase, or the time between two stimuli is too long, the effects of overcompensation will decrease, leading to a process of involution or a phase of little if any improvement in performance capacity.

Following the application of stimulus in training, the organism experiences fatigue (Phase I). During the rest period (Phase II), biochemical stores are not only replenished but exceed normal levels. The organism compensates fully, followed by a rebounding, or over-compensation phase (Phase III), when a higher adaptation occurs, accompanied by a functional increase in athletic efficiency. If another stimulus is not applied at the optimal time (during the overcompensation phase) then involution (decrease in the benefit of overcompensation) occurs (Phase IV).

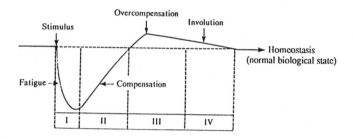

Figure 11. *The overcompensation cycle of a training session (modi-*
fied from Yakovlev, 1967).

Following optimal training stimuli of a training session, the recovery period, including the overcompensation phase, is approximately 24 hours. But variations regarding the occurrence of overcompensation depend on the type and intensity of training. For instance, following a training session to develop aerobic endurance, overcompensation may happen after approximately six hours. High intensity activity, such as plyometric training, which places a high demand on the CNS, may need even more than 24 hours, and sometimes as much as 36 hours for overcompensation to occur.

The strength of various stimuli has a direct effect on the organism's reaction to training. Consequently, as illustrated in Figure 12, a phase in which maximal intensity stimuli (e.g. plyometrics) are overemphasized may lead to a state of general exhaustion and a decrease in performance. This is the typical approach of some overzealous coaches who want to project an image of being "tough" and "hard working", and who, out of ignorance, believe that in each workout the athlete has to reach the state of exhaustion.

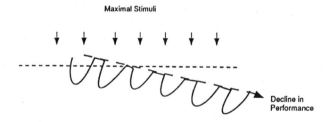

Figure 12. *The decline in performance as a result of exposure to*
prolonged maximal intensity stimuli.

In such circumstances, there is never time to compensate, since the depth of the curve of fatigue sinks deeper, a reality which requires not another "hard" workout, but rather a low-intensity stimuli and time to regenerate. This will result in compensation and ultimately in over-compensation as well.

It is certainly true that in order to constantly improve performance, the coach has to regularly challenge the potential reached by an athlete, in order to continue to elevate the ceiling of adaptation. In practical terms, however, this means that high intensity stimuli have to be planned to alternate with low intensity stimuli, so that days of high intensity training are succeeded by low intensity (or no plyometrics) days. This will enhance compensation, and lead to the desired state of overcompensation (Figure 13).

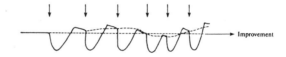

Figure 13. The alternation of maximal and low intensity stimuli produces a wave-like curve of improvement.

TRAINING PRINCIPLES AS APPLIED
TO PLYOMETRIC TRAINING

The process of training is a complex activity, governed by several principles and methodological guidelines. These principles and guidelines assist the coach in selecting the best avenues to higher performance, the methods to be considered, and the best progression to be employed.

Derived from the need to fulfill specific training goals, in this case to improve plyometric power, these principles are part of a conceptual framework and therefore should not be viewed in isolation. However, for the purpose of a more convenient presentation, each principle is presented separately. A thorough comprehension and utilization of these principles will ensure a superior organization of training with the least errors possible.

Principle of Specificity

In order to be effective and lead to the highest adaptation, training has to be aimed specifically at developing the energy system required, to attempt to improve the dominant physical performance factor of a given sport. Similarly, training programs must be relevant to the specific physical demands of the sport/event in which the athlete specializes. From a physiological point of view such demands should refer to:

1) *the dominant energy system.*
   In the case of plyometric training, the energy is provided by the anaerobic alactic and lactic systems.
2) *the specific muscle groups* involved as well as the movement patterns characteristic of the selected sport.

Thus, plyometric exercises have to mimic as much as possible the key movement patterns, the dominant skills of the sport, and improve the power of the prime movers, the muscles required to perform a specific technical movement. Normally, gains in power have a positive transfer to improvement in skill.

In order to attain maximal improvement of the energy system for plyometric training and power for the prime movers, plyometric exercises ought to be carefully selected with specific reasons in mind. Only this selective approach will increase the effectiveness of the fast-twitch muscle fibres which are employed in these exercises.

Another aspect of specificity of training -- at least in strength training--is the fact that improvements are angle specific (Lindh, 1979). This means that if an athlete trains at a certain angle, often typical of isometric training, training effects will be visible at, and around that particular angle. Consequently, it makes physiological sense to train at all the angles, throughout the whole range of motion.

In the case of plyometric training, the only exercises affected by this are the drop (shock) jumps, where the athlete should land, and maintain this position for 1-2 seconds, in a flexed position at a given angle. Varying the angle of the main limbs during landing will certainly compensate for this shortcoming.

"Cross-training", or the transfer of training benefits from one region of the body to another, has been researched since the 1920s. Setchenov (1935) claims that training the right arm resulted in some strength improvements on the other arm as well. Some evidence also exists regarding the transfer from legs to arms. Pollock (1973) concluded that leg exercises did influence the electrical activity, and as such the tension in the muscle, of the arm muscles. Although this research supports the existence of an electro-physiological transfer from one set of limbs to the others, there still does not exist conclusive evidence of either transfer of training effect or maintenance of fitness. Consequently, it is safe to conclude that although some "cross-training" effect may exist, specificity of training ought to be observed in plyometric training as well. All the prime movers employed in the sport should be addressed, regardless of the body part involved.

Principle of Individualization

Individualization in training is one of the main requirements of contemporary training and refers to the fact that each athlete, regardless of the level of performance, must be treated individually according to ability, potential, learning characteristics and specificity of sport. The whole training concept has to be modelled in accordance with the athlete's particular characteristics, so that training objectives may be enhanced appropriately.

Individualization should not be perceived only as a method of correcting individual technical deficiencies, or the specialization of an individual in an event or position played in a team, but rather a means by which an athlete is evaluated objectively and observed subjectively. The coach may then assess the athlete's training needs and maximize the athlete's abilities.

However, much too often, in their quest for easy gains, some coaches slavishly follow training programs of successful athletes, completely disregarding the athlete's particular needs, experience and abilities. What is even worse, such programs are sometimes inserted into junior athletes' training schedules. These athletes are both physiologically and psychologically incapable of following such programs, especially the high intensity components. Therefore, in order to be effective and to maximize the athlete's abilities, particular attention should be paid to the following basic training rules:

- Prior to designing a training program, the coach should analyze the athlete's training potential and personality development, in order to determine the limits of tolerance to work. Often the individual's working capacity depends on the following factors:

  - *Biological and chronological age*, especially for children and juniors whose bodies have not yet reached maturity. Their training, as compared to that of mature athletes, should be of a more complex nature, with plenty of variety and of moderate intensity. Juniors may more readily tolerate a higher volume of training rather than high intensity or heavy loads which can overtax their anatomical structures, especially the bones (which are not ossified yet), ligaments, tendons and muscles.

  - *Training background*, or the age at which the athlete began participation in sports. The work demand should be proportional to the level of experience of the athlete. Although the rate of improvement of some athletes may be different, the coach still has to be cautious with regard to the load which may be undertaken. Similarly, when athletes of different backgrounds and experiences are assigned to train in the same group, the coach should not ignore their individual characteristics and potential.

  - *Individual capacity for work and performance*. Not all athletes who are capable of the same performance have the same work capacity. There are several biological and psychological factors which determine the individual's work abilities.

- *Training and health status.* Training status dictates the content, load and rate of training. Athletes with the same level of performance have different levels of strength, speed, endurance development, and skills. Such dissimilarities justify the need for individualization in training. Furthermore, individualization is strongly recommended for athletes who experience illness or injury. Thus, health status also determines the limits of the individual's training capacity. Such limits and limitations should be known by the coach and only close co-operation between the coach and a physiologist or physician may resolve the problem.

- *Training load and the athlete's rate of recovery.* When planning and evaluating the work in training, the coach must take into consideration factors outside of training which may place a high demand on the athlete. Heavy involvement in school, work, or family, distance to travel to school or training can affect the rate of recovery between training lessons. By the same token, the athlete's lifestyle and emotional involvement should also be known by the coach. These factors must be properly assessed in planning the content and stress of training.

- *The athlete's particular physique* could play an important role in both training load and performance capacity. Individual particularities can be determined through adequate testing, for which the coach may solicit the assistance of appropriate specialists.

- Work adaptation is a function of individual capacity. As far as training programs for children and juniors are concerned, although precise standards regarding training loads are rarely found, young athletes tend to adapt more easily to a higher volume of training with moderate intensity.

- Women's particular anatomical structure and biological differences require specific consideration in the design of plyometric training programs. In general, strength training for women should be rigorously continuous, without long interruptions. As far as plyometric exercises are concerned, a careful progression should be observed over a longer period of time.

- There is a direct relation between the menstrual cycle of female athletes and their physical and psychological efficiency and behaviour. Exercise does not appear to significantly affect menstrual disorders (Matthews and Fox, 1976) but eventually unfavourable changes were observed in younger, rather than in more mature female athletes. During menstruation, younger female athletes

35

should be exposed to training in a progressive manner, and, following an appropriate phase of adaptation to moderate exercises, they may engage in progressively heavier training. In any case, the amount of work should be determined on an individual basis. As far as plyometric training is concerned, exercises such as reactive and drop jumps should be avoided. Experienced athletes, those with a good background in power training, may be exposed to low impact exercises.

Principle of Progressive Increase in Training Load

Improvement of performance is a direct result of the amount and quality of work achieved in training. From the initiation stage right up to the elite performance stage, workload in training has to be increased gradually, in accordance with each individual's physiological and psychological abilities.

The physiological basis of this principle rests on the fact that as a result of training the body's functional efficiency and thereby its capacity to do work gradually increases over a long period of time. Similarly, any drastic increase in one's performance requires a long period of training and adaptation (Astrand and Rodahl, 1986). The body reacts anatomically, physiologically and psychologically to the demands of the increased training load. Consideration must also be given to the fact that improvement in the functions and reactions of the nervous system, in neuro-muscular coordination and the psychological capacity to cope with the stress resulting from heavy training loads, also occurs gradually. The process requires time and competent technical leadership.

The principle of gradual increase of load in training is the basis for all planning of athletic training, and should be followed by all athletes regardless of their level of performance. The rate at which performance improves depends directly on the rate and manner in which the training load is increased. An impediment in the increase of work in training results in stagnation. It also should be noted that repetition of the same standard stimuli (same workload) leads to a dissipation of the training effect. In the long run, this will be reflected in physical and psychological deterioration and a reduction in performance capacity. As illustrated in Figure 14, the result of a standard stimulus is initially evolution, followed by a plateau, and ultimately involution, or a decrease in performance.

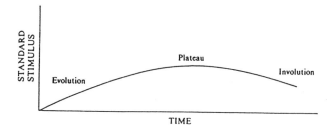

Figure 14. The three phases of the curve resulting from a standard stimulus (similar load employed for a longer period of time).

In the past, several research studies have investigated methods of increasing the work in training. The overloading or the linear and continuous methods were found to be less effective than the step or undulatory approach (Ozolin, 1971; Harre, 1981). In contrast to the linear approach, the step type method fulfils the physiological and psychological requirement that a training load increase must be followed by a phase of unloading during which the organism adapts and regenerates, thus preparing for a new increase. The recurrence of the increase in training load must be determined in accordance with each individual's needs, rate of adaptation and competitive calendar. A very abrupt increase in training load may go beyond the athlete's capacity to adapt, thereby affecting the physiological and especially psychological balance. Ultimately, such an approach may result in symptoms of overtraining and even injuries, especially for athletes following plyometric training programs.

The step-type approach (Figure 15) to elevating the training load should not be interpreted as a steady increase in each training session through the arithmetical addition of equal quantities of work. A training session is insufficient to cause visible changes in the body. To achieve such an adaptation, it is necessary to repeat the same type of training session or training stimulus several times. Often, training sessions of the same type may be planned for an entire week, followed then by another increase in the training load.

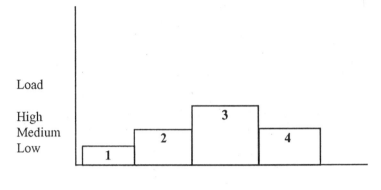

WEEKS (MICROCYCLES)

Figure 15.   The increase of training load in steps.

Figure 15 illustrates how the training load is increased in a macrocycle, which is a phase of training of 2-6 (usually 4) weeks. Each vertical line represents a change in training load while the horizontal line represents the phase of adaptation required by the new demand. The load is increased gradually in the first three microcycles followed by a preparatory decrease or unloading phase, allowing the body to regenerate. The purpose of regeneration is to enable the athlete to accumulate physiological and psychological reserves in anticipation of further increases in the training load. Training performance usually improves following a regeneration phase.

The fourth cycle in this example, the unloading phase, represents the new lowest step for another macrocycle. However, since the body has already adjusted to the previous loads, the new low step is not of the same magnitude as the previous low, but rather equal to the medium one.

An increase in training load produces slight physiological fatigue followed by an adaptation phase during which the organism adjusts to the training demand, culminating in an improvement in performance (or in scheduled tests).

There is a direct relationship between the length and height of the step. The shorter the length of the adaptation phase, the lower the height, or the amount of increase in training load. A longer adaptation phase may allow a higher increase.

Although the increase of training load does progress in steps, in a training plan of longer duration, the training load curve appears to have an undulatory shape, which is enhanced by the continuous alternations of increase and decrease of the components of training (Figure 16).

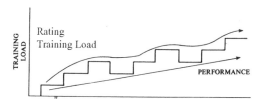

Figure 16. The training load curve appears to be undulatory while the performance improves continuously (the arrow).

The increase in training load should also be governed by the rate of improvement of performance in a sport. The quicker the rate of performance improvement, the greater the training loads required. Otherwise, the athlete never will catch up with contemporary performance.

The magnitude of the training load has to be elevated not only for shorter training cycles, but also from year to year. Both the volume (quantity) and intensity (quality) of training have to be increased each year, otherwise stagnation in performance is inevitable. Therefore the volume of training from year to year could increase anywhere between 20-50%. However, the increase in the number of training sessions has to allow for individual capacity, adaptability, training time, level of performance and the need to alternate constantly varying training intensities.

METHODOLOGICAL GUIDELINES
FOR PLYOMETRIC TRAINING

Among the many methodological factors which are important for the successful application of plyometric training, some of them, such as intensity and rest interval, are crucial. This chapter focuses on these factors.

It is widely recognized that a good background of several years of strength training will assist in advancing faster through the progression of plyometric exercises. This experience is also an important factor in preventing injury. Strength training programs should not revolve only around the legs or arms extensors, but should focus particularly on strengthening the "core" muscles: the abdominals, the lower back, and spinal column musculature. These sets of muscles, (the hips and spine) work together as shock absorbers for plyometric exercises. Consequently, when preparing athletes--especially young ones--for a program of plyometrics, the coach should start from the core section of the body and work towards the extremities. In other words, before strengthening the legs and arms, concentrate on developing the link between them, the support, which is the spinal column, using exercises such as back extensions, side bending, hip flexion and extension against low resistance.

As far as establishing a good base of strength and developing shock-absorbing qualities are concerned, the benefits of introducing children to plyometric exercises should not be dismissed, providing these exercises are performed over a period of several years, and the principle of progression is respected (Figure 18). The key element of this approach is PATIENCE. A healthy training progression would be to expose children to low impact plyometrics first, during a period of several years, say between the ages of 14 and 16 years, and only after that introduce the young athlete to the more demanding reactive jumps.

Throughout these years of a long-term progression, teachers in the school system and coaches in sports clubs should teach young athletes the correct plyometric techniques, in which the "hop" and "step" from the triple jump are the ABC of plyometric training.

In addition to the amount of strength which should be developed before doing plyometrics (some authors consider the ability to perform half squats with a load of twice the body weight is a safe guide), the type of training surface, the equipment to wear, and whether to carry additional weights when performing plyometric exercises (heavy vests, ankle and waist belts) are also controversial topics.

For the person concerned about injury, the surface of the floor should be soft. That means that outdoors these exercises should be performed on grass or soft ground, and indoors on a padded floor. Although this precaution may be appropriate for beginners, it should be remembered that a soft surface could dampen the stretch reflex. Only a solid surface can enhance the reactivity of the neuro-muscular system. Therefore, for athletes with a better background in sports and/or strength training, a solid surface is recommended. The training surface is not the only important element to consider in order to avoid injuries, but rather to follow a very methodical progression over several years of training.

Footwear is also a contentious issue and there seem to be two completely different approaches, the East European and the North American. European athletes--even young ones--very often perform many exercises barefoot (see Figure 17) and they run, jump, and play on grass and sand, barefoot.

The major argument put forward by East European physicians is based on the view that a free foot, without the support given by shoes or tape, will better develop the ligaments and tendons of the foot. In this way the probability of injuries is much lower.

North Americans, on the other hand, always wear athletic shoes. In most cases, they do not play games without taping the ankles. However, the European view is that the tape represents an artificial support, which does not enhance the natural way of strengthening the ligaments, tendons, and the ankle joint in general. In any case, the traditional North American approach is to wear shoes for plyometric exercises, with a good sole and ankle support.

Finally, weighted ankle and waist belts should not be used during plyometric drills, simply because (as in the case of a soft surface) they help to decrease the reactive ability of the nerve-muscle coupling and obstruct the reactivity of the neuro-muscular system.

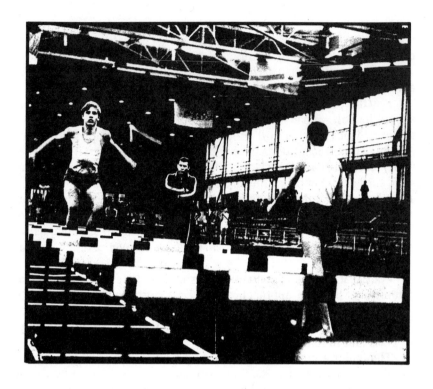

Figure 17. A plyometric session with young track athletes in Russia.

Furthermore, while such overloading may result in increased strength, it certainly slows down the speed of reaction and rebounding effect.

Intensity and Classificaton of Intensities in Plyometrics

The level of intensity is directly proportional to the height and/or length of an exercise. High intensity plyometric exercises, such as reactive or drop jumps, result in higher tension in the muscle, recruiting more neuro-muscular units to perform the action or to resist the pull of gravitational force.

Plyometric exercises can be divided into two major groups, reflecting the degree of impact the exercises have on the neuro-muscular system:

1. LOW IMPACT EXERCISES:
- skipping
- rope jumps
- jumps: low and short steps, hops and jumps
- jumps over low benches/ rope: 10-15" (25-35 cm)
- medicine ball throws: 5-9lbs (2-4kg)
- tubing
- throwing of light implements (i.e. baseball)

2. HIGH IMPACT EXERCISES:
- standing long, and triple jump
- jumps: higher and longer steps, hops and jumps
- jumps over higher benches/ rope: >15" (35 cm)
- jumps on, over, and off boxes of >15" (35 cm)
- heavy medicine ball throws: 11-13lbs (5-6kg)
- throwing heavy implements
- drop jumps/reactive jumps
- "shock" muscle tension induced by machines

From a more practical perspective, plyometric exercises can be divided into five groups of intensity (see Figure 18). As discussed in the chapter on planning (Chapter 7), this classification can be utilized to facilitate better alternation of training demand throughout the week.

Any plan to incorporate plyometric exercises into a training program should consider the following factors:
- the age and physical development of the athlete
- the skills and techniques involved in plyometric exercises
- the principal performance factors of the sport
- the energy requirements of the sport
- the particular training phase of the annual plan
- the need to respect a methodical progression over a longer period of time (2-4 years): to progress from low impact (#5 and #4) to simple bounding (#3), and then to high impact exercises (#2 and #1).

Plyometric exercises are fun to perform but because they demand a high level of concentration, they are deceptively vigorous and taxing. The lack of patience and discipline to wait for the right moment for each exercise can result in incorporating high impact exercises into the training program of athletes who are still not ready. Often, the resultant injuries or physiological discomfort is not the fault of the plyometric exercises themselves, but rather the lack of knowledge and application of the coach or instructor.

Intensity Values #	Type of Exercise	Intensity of Exercise	No. of Reps/ and Sets	No. of Reps/ Training Session	Rest Interval Between Sets
1	Shock Tension High Reactive Jumps >25'(>60cm)	Maximal	8-5 x 10-20	120 -150 (200)	8 - 10 min.
2	Drop Jumps >35-48 (80-120 cm)	Very High	5-15 x 5-15	75-100	5-7 min.
3	Bounding Exercises -2 legs -1 leg	Submaximal	3-25 x 5-15	50-250	3-5 min.
4	Low Reactive Jumps 8-20' (20-50 cm)	Moderate	10-25 x10-25	150-250	3-5 min.
5	Low Impact Jumps/Throws -On Spot -Implements	Low	10-30 x10-15	50-300	2 -3 min.

Figure 18. The five levels of intensity of plyometric exercises.

This is why knowledge of the five levels of intensity will help in the selection of appropriate exercises and rest interval. However, the suggested number of repetitions and sets are for advanced athletes. The coach should resist the temptation to apply the same number of repetitions and sets to beginners, or athletes with insufficient foundation in sports and/or strength training.

Progress through the five degrees of intensity is a long-term proposition. The incorporation of low impact exercises into the training program of young athletes, for 2-4 years, represents the time needed for a progressive adaptation of ligaments, tendons, and the bony structure of the limbs involved. It also allows for the gradual preparation of the shock-absorbing sections of the body, such as the hips and spine.

Figure 19 illustrates a long-term, comprehensive progression of strength and power training, including plyometric training. It is important to observe the age at which it is suggested that low-impact plyometrics be introduced, and the fact that high-impact plyometrics are only introduced after four years. This implies that this is the length of time required to learn proper technique and to allow for a progressive anatomical adaptation. From this point on in the athlete's training, high impact plyometrics could be part of the normal diet of training.

The intensity in plyometric exercises--the amount of tension created in the muscle--depends on the height of the exercise performed. Although the height is determined strictly by the individual qualities of the athlete, the following general principle applies: the stronger the muscular system the greater the energy required to stretch it to obtain an elastic effect in the shortening phase. This is why optimal height for one athlete may not generate the greatest stimulation for another. Therefore, the following information should be treated only as guidelines.

According to Verkhoshanski (1968) the optimal height for depth (reactive) jumps for speed training is between 30 inches (75cm) and 43 inches (110cm), in order to make gains in dynamic strength (power). Similar findings were reported by Katschajov et al. (1976), and Bosco and Komi (1980). Above 43 inches, the latter authors concluded, the mechanics of the action are changed, so that the time and energy it takes to cushion the force of the drop on the ground defeats the purpose of plyometric training. Exceptional heights were tried by other authors: Zanon (1977) employed the following heights for international class long jumpers: 8.2 feet (2.50m) for men, and 7 feet (2.10m) for women. The landing from boxes of these heights was immediately followed by a long jump for distance!

Age Groups	Forms of Training	Methods	Volume	Intensity	Means of Training
NOVICE 12 - 13	- general exercises only - games	- muscular endurance	- low - medium	- very low	- light resistance exercises - light implements - medicine balls - balls
BEGINNERS 13 - 15	- general strength - event oriented exercises	- muscular endurance - introduce low impact plyometrics	- low - medium - high	- low	- **dumb-bells** - tubing - medicine balls - universal gym.
INTERMEDIATE 15-17	- general strength - event oriented	- body building - circuit training (muscular endurance) - power - low impact plyometrics	as above	- low - medium	- all the above - free weights
ADVANCED >17	- event oriented - specific strength	- body building - muscle endurance - power - max. strength - low impact plyometrics - introduce high impact plyometrics	- medium - high - maximal	- medium - high	- free weights - special strength/power equipment
HIGH PERFORMANCE	- specific	- all the above - eccentric - plyometrics - low impact - high impact	as above	- medium - high - super max.	as above

Figure 19. A long-term strength development and the progression of plyometric training.

The Number of Repetitions and Sets

As far as the number of repetitions is concerned, plyometric exercises fall into two categories: single-response (SR) and multiple-response (MR) drills. The former as illustrated by Figure 18 represents a single action such as high reactive jumps, shock tension (#1), and drop jumps (#2) where the main purpose is to induce the highest level of tension in the muscles. The objective of such exercises is to develop maximum strength and power. The repetitive exercises such as bounding (#3), low reactive (#4), and low impact (#5) result in the development of power and power endurance. Therefore, as suggested in Figure 18, the number of repetitions could be anywhere between 1 and 30, with the number of sets ranging from 5-25, depending on the scope of training, type of exercise, and the athlete's background and physical potential.

Often, however, especially for MR exercises, it is more convenient and practical to equate the numbers of repetitions with a distance, e.g. 5 sets of 50m rather than 5 sets of 25 repetitions. In this way, it is not necessary to constantly count the number of repetitions.

The Rest Interval Between Sets

One of the factors for high-quality training is adequate physiological recuperation between exercises.

Far too often athletes/coaches either do not pay enough attention to the duration of the rest interval, or are simply caught up in the "traditions" of a given sport. Quite often "tradition" dictates that the only rest interval taken is the time necessary to move from one station to another. There is no question that this is quite inadequate, especially when the physiological characteristics of plyometric training are taken into consideration.

The fatigue induced by plyometric exercises is twofold: local, and fatigue affecting the Central Nervous System (CNS). Local fatigue is experienced as a result of depleting the energy stored in the muscle, the fuel necessary to perform such explosive movements (CP and ATP), and the production of lactic acid for repetitions longer than 10-15 seconds.

But even more important, during training athletes are fatiguing the CNS, the very system which is determinant in sending powerful signals to the working muscle to perform a given amount of quality work. This is why, in the last few years, power and strength training with loads of more than 70% of maximum has been called "nervous system training", as a way of acknowledging the importance of the CNS in high quality training.

Plyometric training is performed as a result of nerve impulses sent by the CNS to the working muscle. These impulses have a certain speed, power, and frequency. Any high quality training requires that the speed of contraction, its power, or frequency, be at the highest level possible.

When the rest interval is short (1-2 minutes), the athlete experiences both local and CNS fatigue. For the working muscle, a short rest interval means the inability to remove the lactic acid from the muscle, and to replenish the energy necessary to perform the next repetitions with the same intensity. Similarly, a fatigued CNS is no longer able to send the powerful nerve impulses which ensure that the prescribed load is performed with the same number of repetitions and sets before exhaustion is experienced. And from exhaustion to injury is often just a short step! Therefore maximum attention should be paid to the rest interval!

As suggested in Figure 18, the rest interval is a function of the load and type of plyometric training performed. The higher the intensity of the exercise, the greater the rest interval. Consequently, for maximal intensity (high reactive jumps) the rest interval between sets should be 8-10 minutes, or even longer. The suggested rest for intensity #2 is 5-7 minutes, for #3 and #4 between 3-5 minutes, while for low impact activities (#5) around 2-3 minutes.

PLANNING

Like most complex human endeavours, training must be well organized and planned in order to ensure the achievement of training objectives. Thus, the planning process in training represents a methodical and scientific procedure which assists the athlete to achieve the desired performance. Consequently, planning is the most important tool utilized by the coach in attempting to conduct a well-organized training program. A coach is only as efficient as he or she is organized. A plyometric training program is successful only if it is well-designed, based on the scientific knowledge available in this field, and if it considers periodization of strength as the key guideline to plan strength and power training throughout the year.

The compilation of a plan, both short and long-term, also reflects the coach's knowledge of methodology, and takes appropriate account of the athlete's background and physical potential.

A training plan has to be simple, objective, and above all flexible, as its contents may have to be modified to match the athlete's rate of adaptation to the physiological challenges and improvements in performance.

In this chapter, the reader will be exposed to several types of plans, from the single training session to the long-term. Since planning theory is very complex, and since in this book planning is referred to as it pertains only to plyometric training, for further information on this topic, please refer to the book *Theory and Methodology of Training* (Bompa, 1990).

The Training Session Plan

The training session could be described as the main tool utilized to organize the daily program. For better management and organization, the training session can be structured in four main segments.

The Introduction

The session begins with a discussion with the athletes of the training objectives for the day, and how they are going to be achieved. At the same time the coach can use certain methods to challenge and motivate the athletes for the work to be done. If parts of the program have to be performed in groups, the coach will divide the athletes at this point, giving them the appropriate information and guidelines.

The Physiological Preparation for Training
The Warm Up

The warm-up is a subject of controversy among many researchers. However, most of them agree that warm-up facilitates performance and prepares the athlete physically and mentally for the training tasks ahead. A warm-up is necessary in order to elevate the athlete's efficiency from a resting state. Therefore, the role of the warm-up is to reach a state of high physiological efficiency prior to the beginning of a competition or the main part of the training session.

During the warm-up, body temperature is raised, which appears to be one of the main factors facilitating performance. Moreover, the warm-up stimulates the activity of the CNS which coordinates all the systems of the body, speeds up motor reactions through faster transmission of nerve impulses, and improves coordination. Also, by elevating the body temperature, muscles, tendons, ligaments and other tissues are warmed-up and stretched, thereby preventing and/or reducing ligament sprains, and tendon and muscle strains. The warm-up also allows the athlete to focus on and to prepare psychologically for the task ahead. During warm-up the athlete activates and prepares most of the proprioceptors and establishes neuro-muscular patterns of performance by repeating parts of the training routine or skills. Warm-up is composed of two parts: the general warm-up, and the specific warm-up.

General Warm-Up

The purpose of the general warm-up is to elevate the body's work capacity, by increasing body temperature, so that the athlete can perform more effectively. As a result of elevated body temperature, the blood flow increases along with the rate of metabolism, which in turn stimulates the respiratory centre, leading to an increase in the oxygen supply available to the body. The best way to warm up the body is to perform a series of physical exercises. A warm-up should be progressive from low to moderate intensity, and of longer duration. In order to determine the optimal duration, body temperature should be checked, or alternatively, the onset of perspiration signifies that the desired body temperature has been reached and marks the end of the warm-up. Generally speaking, the duration of the warm-up should be between 20-

30 minutes, or longer. However, it depends on the athlete's physical preparation, general endurance and the ambient environmental temperature. For a long distance runner a 10-minute run for a warm-up is not sufficient, but it might be enough for a sprinter. Also, it will take a longer time for an athlete to warm up and to begin to perspire in a cold environment as opposed to a warm environment. For example, when the external environmental temperature is 8°C (46° Fahrenheit) perspiration may start after 12-13 minutes of uninterrupted work. In a warm environment, an intensive, uninterrupted warm-up may yield the same results after 2-3 minutes. However that may not be enough time to reach full functional potential.

Warm-up exercises should be performed at lower speed than in training or competition, and they should be very similar or identical to the skills to be performed. The frequency and number of repetitions of exercises or skills must be adjusted according to the environmental temperature, specifics of the sport, and the athlete's level of physical preparation.

A warm-up should start with slow running of various forms (sideways, backwards, but mostly forward) for 5-10 minutes, followed by calisthenics and stretching exercises. Calisthenic exercises may be performed from top to bottom, starting with neck, arms and shoulder, abdomen, legs and back. Stretching exercises for flexibility should not be done prior to running since they do not generate blood flow in the way that running does. Also, cold muscles are harder to stretch and easily injured. Flexibility exercises may be followed by some light jumping or bounding exercises, if it is appropriate to the sport. A few short sprints (20-40m) may complete the general warm-up. Rest and muscle relaxation (shaking the limbs) between all these exercises should be included, so that the athlete is sure of completing a relaxing and not overly demanding warm-up. During the warm-up the athlete should also prepare mentally and psychologically for the main part of the training session or competition, by trying to visualize the skills to be performed and thereby providing motivation to perform the more difficult aspects of the skills.

Specific Warm-Up

The main objective of the specific warm-up is to get the athlete ready for the type of work to be performed during the main part of the training session. This preparation phase includes mental preparation, coordination of certain exercises, preparation of the CNS and consequently elevation of the body's working capacity.

The exercises performed during a specific warm-up depend on the type of exercises and skills to be performed in the main part of the session or competition. A gymnast, wrestler, figure skater, thrower or jumper may perform certain technical elements or parts of a routine; a swimmer, runner or rower may repeat starts or wind sprints with the rhythm and intensity close or similar to the main part of the training session or competition. A specific warm-up should be performed by every athlete, especially by those whose skills are very complex. The more complex the skill is, the more it should be repeated. The duration of the specific warm-up depends on the volume of work to be performed, and on the duration of the competition. The greater the volume of work or the longer the competition, the longer the warm-up should be.

The warm-up is an important component of training. To warm-up properly requires good general physical preparation and general endurance. Only fit athletes can perform a 20-30 minute warm-up. In fact, warm-up is utilized as a way of developing general physical fitness, especially during the preparatory season.

If plyometric exercises are to be performed immediately following the specific warm-up, then the coach can expose the athletes to a few progressively demanding drills.

The Main Part of the Training Session

This part of the session is dedicated to actual training, performing the drills, skills, and tactics planned for that particular day. As far as the content of the training session is concerned, the sequence of exercises should be based on the state of the CNS and how it may affect learning or the acquisition of certain abilities. The following suggested order of events is based on this principle:

1. First the athletes should be exposed to drills which have the goal of learning and/or perfecting technical or tactical elements. Learning is enhanced when the CNS is rested. On the other hand, the incorporation of skill acquisition drills following other activities will affect learning, simply because retention is impeded by fatigue.
2. Plan activities destined to develop speed, reaction, and coordination. Since these types of activities, especially speed and reaction, are affected by the quality of nerve impulses sent by the nervous system to the working muscle, it is strongly advised that such exercises should be performed as early as possible in

the session. Ideally, they should be done immediately following the warm-up, when the athlete is still very fresh, or relatively rested.

3. Exercises aimed at developing strength/power ought to be placed after movements designed to enhance technique or develop speed. The reason is twofold: on the one hand speed/reaction exercises represent an activation of CNS, favourable to strength/power development; on the other hand, on a short-term basis, employing heavy loads first, may impair the development of speed.

4. Finally, the development of endurance has to be placed at the end of the session, since such activity is very demanding and therefore tiring. Obviously, under these conditions, it is not appropriate to expect athletes to acquire skills or develop qualities requiring high velocity and fast reactions.

The inclusion of plyometric exercises in a training session should take into consideration the above realities, the phase of training, but, more importantly, their significance on that day. For instance if power development through the use of plyometrics is the main focus of the day, they have to be placed immediately following the warm-up. Below, the reader will find several options in which plyometrics have to be planned along with other activities. In these examples, plyometrics are considered as the secondary objective of the training session:

#1	#2	#3	#4
Warm-up	Warm-up	Warm-up	Warm-up
Technique	Speed	Technique	Technique
Speed	Plyometrics	Plyometrics	Plyometrics
Plyometrics	Endurance	Endurance	Strength

Certainly, the training load of plyometric exercises has to take into account the physiological and psychological fatigue resulting from the attempt to achieve the main training objective of the day.

The above options do not exhaust all the possibilities. However, it would not be advisable to perform plyometric exercises following endurance or maximum strength work, since the resulting fatigue would impair the reactivity of the nervous system, the stretching-shortening cycle.

The Mycrocycle

A microcycle refers to a weekly training program, and is probably the most important tool in planning. Throughout the annual plan the nature and dynamics of microcycles alternate according to the phase of training, the training objectives, and the physiological and psychological demands of training.

The decision on the order of the type of training session within the microcycle should respect the same physiological concepts and sequence outlined above:

1. Technical and/or tactical elements
2. Speed and/or power
3. Strength
4. Aerobic endurance/muscular endurance.

Often, in order to achieve a training effect, training sessions of similar objectives and content must be repeated 2-3 times during the same microcycle. The repetition of similar exercises several times is imperative for learning a technical skill or developing a biomotor ability. However, during a microcycle, exercises designed to develop motor abilities have to be repeated with varying frequencies. Thus, the development of general endurance, flexibility, or strength in a small muscle group is more effective when it is repeated daily. On the other hand, strength exercises designated for a larger muscle group produce better results when they are repeated every second day. Strength training of larger muscle groups has a cardio-vascular component which is more exhausting and therefore requires a longer recovery period, compared to smaller muscle groups where the training effects are localized. As for the development of specific endurance of submaximal intensity, three training sessions per week will suffice, while specific endurance of maximal intensity during the competitive phase should be planned for two sessions a week with the remaining days being devoted to lower intensity training. Similarly, two sessions per week are adequate for the maintenance of strength, flexibility and speed. Finally, an optimal frequency for plyometric exercises utilized to develop leg power and exercise for speed, performed under strenuous conditions, is 2-3 times per week.

The concept of repeating the same training session 2-3 times during a week of training may also be valid for the microcycles themselves, especially during the preparatory phase. A microcycle of the same nature (i.e., content, methods, etc.) may be repeated 2-3 times, following which improvement based on the adaptation of the body to training may be observed. However, particularly for advanced athletes, the nature of the microcycle may be constant, but the volume and intensity of training should be increased for each cycle.

From the point of view of intensity of training, microcycles follow the principle of the progressive increase of the training load (Figure 20).

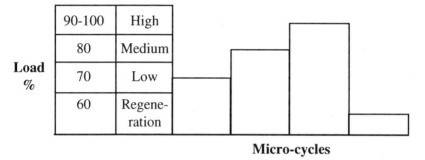

Micro-cycles

Figure 20.   The dynamics of increasing the training load over four microcycles.

As illustrated in Figure 20, during the first three cycles, the load is progressively increased, followed by a regeneration cycle, where the load is decreased, in order to facilitate recuperation and replenishment of energy, and to overcompensate before another load increment of 3-4 microcycles.

The number of days planned for reactive training varies according to the intensity of the microcycle. During a week of low intensity, 1-2 days for plyometric exercises can be planned, say Tuesday and Thursday or Friday. In the second cycle the number of days could increase to 2-3, while in the third week, three reactive training days could be planned. During the regeneration week, there should be one or no plyometric session. The dynamics of the training load also vary within a microcycle. Figures 21 - 23 illustrate three examples.

Planning the plyometric exercises within a microcycle depends on the training phase (see the Annual Plan), the level of intensity, and the characteristics of the sport. In a sport where power is a determinant performance factor, plyometric training will be an important component in training.

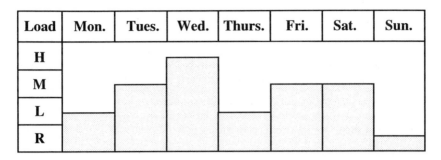

Figure 21. A low intensity microcycle (first level as per Figure 15) where there is one high intensity training day (H), and several medium (M) and low (L) intensity days. Sunday is a rest day (R).

Load	Mon.	Tues.	Wed.	Thurs.	Fri.	Sat.	Sun.
H							
M							
L							
R							

Figure 22. An example of a medium intensity microcycle (second level as per Figure 15).

Load	Mon.	Tues.	Wed.	Thurs.	Fri.	Sat.	Sun.
H							
M							
L							
R							

Figure 23. A high intensity microcycle (third level as per Figure 15) where three high intensity training days are planned.

56

The actual planning of plyometric training for a microcycle should follow the five intensity levels proposed in Figure18. The utilization of these intensity levels will allow the coach to alternate various kinds of plyometrics, so that the athlete is not always taxed to the same extent throughout the week. Similarly, in making such changes, the coach should consider the overcompensation concept. Therefore, training days resulting in a high level of fatigue should alternate with low level days, which will facilitate the occurrence of overcompensation with all its physiological benefits.

Figures 24 and 25 illustrate the practicality of employing the five intensity levels, as well as how the overcompensation concept reacts to the dynamics of altering these intensities.

In the first example, note that the lowest levels of fatigue are triggered by intensity levels #1 and #2. This is illustrated by the depth of the fatigue curves. Similarly, after this kind of training day, there is no overcompensation, illustrated by the fact that the curve does not reach the homeostasis level (the interrupted horizontal line). Overcompensation is experienced two days later, before the training sessions on Thursday, Saturday and Sunday.

A similar trend is seen in Figure 25, where the three high intensity plyometric sessions are planned for Tuesday, Thursday, and Saturday. The physiological reaction--a high level of fatigue--is to be expected. However, since these demanding sessions are planned 48 hours apart, overcompensation may occur just in time, before the next demanding training session.

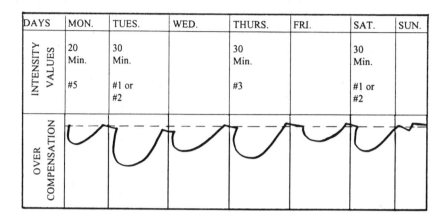

DAYS	MON.	TUES.	WED.	THURS.	FRI.	SAT.	SUN.
INTENSITY VALUES	20 Min. #5	30 Min. #1 or #2		30 Min. #3		30 Min. #1 or #2	
OVER COMPENSATION							

Figure 24. A hypothetical example of a micro-cycle where two highly intensive plyometric exercises are planned, illustrated by the depth of the fatigue curves. Similarly, following such days of training, one does not overcompensate, illustrated by the fact that the curve did not reach the homeostasis level (the interrupted horizontal line). Overcompensation is experienced two days later, before the training session on Thursday and Saturday and Sunday.

DAYS	MON.	TUES.	WED.	THURS.	FRI.	SAT.	SUN.
INTENSITY VALUES	20 Min. #5	30 Min. #1 or #2		20 Min. #3 or #4	30 Min. #1 or #2		OFF
OVER-COMPENSATION							

Figure 25. An example of a micro-cycle where three highly intensive plyometric exercises are planned.

Certainly, in most cases, plyometric exercises are planned on the same days as other activities such as technical and/or tactical work are performed. Similarly, in a training session a coach may plan to work on the development of certain physical qualities such as speed, strength or endurance. Then what is the best approach to be considered in planning plyometric training?

Some authors (Radcliffe and Farentinos, 1985) and coaches suggest that reactive training should be planned for "easy days." To a certain extent, this makes sense. However, from a physiological point of view, this issue demands a more complex interpretation.

Most sports need to train, to a greater or lesser extent, most, if not all of the motor abilities (speed, strength, endurance). Each capacity is dependent on and utilizes a certain energy system. But the recovery, overcompensation, and replenishment of the fuel utilized by each energy system has a different rate. For instance, following aerobic training, overcompensation is reached in approximately 6-8 hours. The same dynamics are not true for speed and power. The recovery or overcompensation from high intensity activities is a minimum of 24 hours which in fact corresponds to the time necessary for the glycogen overcompensation cycle to be completed (Brooks et al., 1973). Following training of maximal intensity, as evidenced by the sprinting program followed by Ben Johnson, it sometimes took up to 48 hours before overcompensation was experienced. Consequently, the days when plyometric training is planned are the days for training speed or power. In this way the athlete depletes the energy system utilized during the training session and does not interfere with the days when other energy systems are taxed. Therefore, if on an "easy day" the athlete also performs plyometric exercises, and on the following days speed or power training, that means that the anaerobic alactic and lactic systems, using glycogen as a fuel, are taxed every single day without allowing the possibility of replenishing the depleted fuel (which requires at least 24 hours). Based on this physiological notion, Figure 26 illustrates a practice which is highly questionable, while Figure 27 represents a combination which allows each energy system and fuel to be replenished and overcompensation to occur.

Further discussion on this topic must also refer to fatigue, and what it is and how it is produced.

For activities of very high intensity and short duration, such as plyometric exercises, the immediate sources of energy for muscular contraction are ATP and CP. Complete depletion of these two chemical components would certainly limit the ability of the muscle to contract (Karlsson and Sahlin, 1971).

Date	Mon.	Tues.	Wed.	Thurs.	Fri.	Sat.	Sun.
Type of Training	Tech-nique Speed	Plyomet-rics Endur-ance	Tech-nique Power	Plyomet-rics Endur-ance	Tech-nique Speed	Tech-nique Power	Off

Figure 26. Planning plyometric exercises on "easy days" is in fact taxing the same energy stores every day without allowing them to be replenished.

Date	Mon.	Tues.	Wed.	Thurs.	Fri.	Sat.	Sun.
Type of Training	Tech-nique Speed Plyomet-rics	Tactical Endur-ance	Tech-nique Plyomet-rics Max. Strength	Tactical Endur-ance	Tech-nique Speed Plyomet-rics	Endur-ance	Off

Figure 27. A planning alternative which facilitates the overcompensation of each energy system.

From the point of view of the energy systems, fatigue occurs when the creatine phosphate is depleted in the working muscle, when muscle glycogen is consumed, or when the carbohydrate store is exhausted as well. The end result is obvious: the work performed by the muscle is decreased, the possible reason being that in a glycogen-depleted muscle, the ATP is produced at a lower rate than it is consumed. Several studies show that carbohydrate is essential to the ability of a muscle to maintain peak force and that endurance capabilities during prolonged, moderate-to-heavy physical activity is directly related to the amount of glycogen in the muscle prior to exercise. This indicates that fatigue occurs as a result of muscle glycogen depletion (Bergstrom et al., 1967). Therefore the above proposal to plan the program based on the energy systems should be considered.

Another argument used by some coaches to plan plyometric exercises on "easy days" is the potential for injury brought about as a result of overtaxing the legs. However, this topic is also very complex, since injuries occur not necessarily as a result of local muscular fatigue (e.g. tired legs) but rather when the whole human machine, especially the CNS is fatigued.

The Annual Plan

The annual plan is the pre-eminent tool for the coach to direct and guide athletic training over a twelve-month period. It is based on the concept of periodization and the principles of training. A training program organized and planned over a year is a necessary requirement in order to maximize improvement in performance.

As was previously stated, the main objective of training is to reach a high level of performance at a given time which usually is the main competition of the year. In order to achieve such a performance, the entire training program has to be properly periodized and planned, so that the development of skills, motor abilities and psychological traits proceeds in a logical and methodical manner.

Periodization is the process of dividing the annual plan into shorter phases of training covering more manageable segments of time, and to ensure correct peaking for the main competition(s) during the year. Such a division enhances appropriate organization of training, allowing the coach to conduct the program in a systematic manner.

The annual training cycle, in most sports, is conventionally divided into three main phases of training: preparation, competition, and transition. Each training phase is further subdivided into cycles, the microcycle being the most important. The duration of each training

61

phase depends heavily on the schedule of competitions, the need to improve skills, and to develop the dominant motor abilities. During the preparatory phase, the coach usually attempts to develop the functional foundations of the athlete's systems, whereas throughout the competitive phase the coach strives for perfection in accordance with the specific demands of competition.

As the reader may be aware, each competition and for that matter the highly intensive training which is specific to the competitive phase, has a strong component of stress. Although most athletes and coaches may cope well with stress, any phase of stressful activities should not be very long. There is a need in training to alternate phases of stressful activities with periods of recovery and regeneration, during which the athletes are exposed to much less pressure. Such a phase (usually the transition phase) facilitates the creation of a favourable mood and regenerates the athlete's potential, thus providing a solid basis for a subsequent period of heavy work.

The Periodization of Strength

Although power is the dominant factor in many sports, training for power (including several types of plyometric exercises throughout the year, from early preparatory to the competitive phase) does not necessarily result in achieving the best results. On the contrary, when the load and type of work performed throughout the year does not alter significantly, it is only at the start that such training represents a stimulus and results in power improvement. As the same type of work is continued in the following phases, the neuro-muscular system adapts to it. If no additional challenge is added, improvement levels off, and so does performance, which may even decline prior to the main competition.

Power is a combined quality: it is the product of gains in maximum strength and speed. In order to improve the level of power from year to year, both maximum strength and speed have to improve as well. However, there are greater genetic limitations to the improvement of speed than to the development of maximum strength, so, of the two factors, more time should be invested in improving maximal strength, the final outcome being the improvement of power.

The dynamics of developing power follows the periodization of strength (Bompa, 1983). Figure 28 illustrates the main phases of strength development, leading to the highest levels of power, or power-endurance.

Preparatory		Competitive		Transition
Anatomical Adaptation	Maximum Strength	Conversion to Power/ Power- Endurance	Maintenance of Power/ Power- Endurance	General Strength

Figure 28. The periodization of strength

Anatomical Adaptation. As the term suggests, during this phase the objective of the training program is to bring about adaptation of the ligaments, tendons and muscle tissue to a progressively increasing training load. In addition, for sports requiring it, muscle mass is also slightly enlarged. Stressless circuit training and a modified body-building method (without working out to exhaustion) could be the main training methods to use. The load should be submaximal (65-80%). Depending on the schedule of competitions and the athlete's classification, the duration of this phase could be anywhere between 4-12 weeks. For experienced athletes, 4-5 weeks will suffice.

Maximum Strength Training has the objective of adapting the neuro-muscular system to heavy loads and fast recruitment of the fast twitch muscle fibres. Since most athletic activities are performed at high speed, even the application of force against heavy loads ought to be exerted as fast as possible. Variations of the weight training method using maximal loads (70-100%) could be considered for a period of 6-12 weeks.

During the *Conversion To Power Phase*, gains in maximum strength should be converted into power or power-endurance. By employing lighter loads, fast contraction, medicine ball throws, and plyometric exercises (intensity levels #3, #4, and #5), the athlete is exposed to activities in which nervous system activation and speed of contraction, are identical to the competitive movements.

Maintenance of Power or power-endurance has to be organized for the duration of the competitive phase. Failing to do so will result in detraining, or the deterioration of the level of power achieved previously. As the physiological basis of performance declines (in this case, power), so does performance and results in competition fall below expectations.

The practical application of the periodization of strength varies in accordance with the type of annual plan, the schedule of competitions, and the classification of the athletes involved. Four different annual plans are presented below. Figure 29 exemplifies an annual plan with only one competitive phase (or mono-cycle, with only one main peak). Both the periodization of strength and plyometric training are presented and then briefly discussed. The second chart, Figure 30, refers to similar topics but for a bi-cycle, or an annual plan with two major peaks per year. The following two figures show examples of two plans: one for a junior athlete (Figure 31), and the other for an international class performer (Figure 32).

On both Figure 29 and 30, below the dates of the plan, the periodization of strength is presented (the classic sequence of Anatomical Adaptation, Maximum Strength, Conversion to Power, Maintenance; and during the Transition phase, General Strength, where the athlete performs basic strength exercises involving most muscle groups). Below that, low impact (intensity levels #5 and #4) and high impact plyometrics (intensity levels#1-3) are indicated.

The solid line shows when a particular kind of plyometric exercise is dominant. Following a basic anatomical adaptation of six weeks, low impact plyometric exercises are introduced progressively. Following 10 weeks of anatomical adaptation and low impact plyometrics (mid Oct.-end of Jan.), from the latter part of January on, high impact plyometric exercises are introduced. The strain of high impact plyometrics is alleviated by alternating two types of exercises (one week of high impact with one week of low impact plyometric exercises). Throughout the maintenance phase, both kinds of plyometrics are utilized to maintain power. This is illustrated by the dotted line.

The two types of plyometric training are planned for specific training objectives. Usually, low impact is aimed at maintaining nervous activation, while high impact has several objectives, such as: maintenance and maximum strength (drop jumps), to shorten the stretching-shortening cycle (reactive jumps), and nervous system peaking. The latter will be referred to at the end of this section on annual planning.

Figure 31 exemplifies a condensed version of annual planning for a junior athlete. The dates of the program are written in such a way that it could refer either to a sport where the competitive phase is in the summer (such as baseball, track, soccer, etc.) or during the winter months (skiing, basketball, volleyball, etc.).

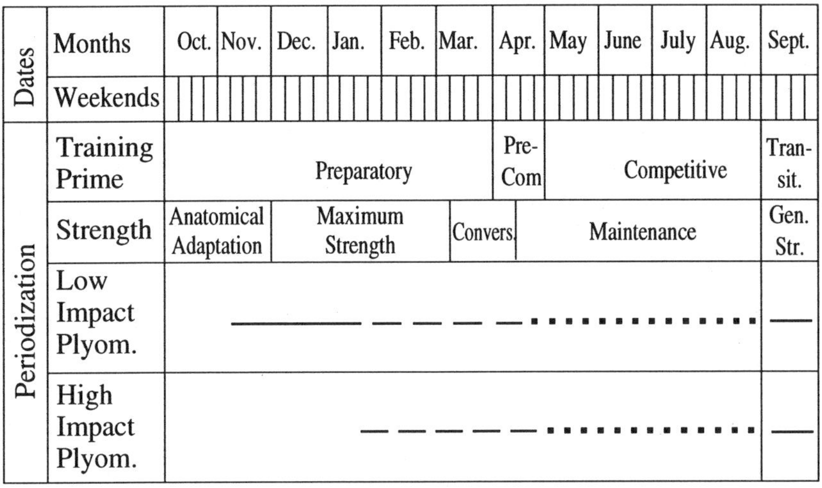

Figure 29 — Annual plan (mono-cycle)

	Months	Oct.	Nov.	Dec.	Jan.	Feb.	Mar.	Apr.	May	June	July	Aug.	Sept.
Dates	Weekends	‖‖‖‖	‖‖‖	‖‖‖	‖‖‖	‖‖‖	‖‖‖	‖‖	‖‖	‖‖‖	‖‖‖	‖‖	‖‖
Periodization	Training Prime	Preparatory						Pre-Com	Competitive				Tran-sit.
	Strength	Anatomical Adaptation		Maximum Strength			Convers.	Maintenance					Gen. Str.
	Low Impact Plyom.												
	High Impact Plyom.												

Figure 29. *An example of an annual plan with only one competitive phase (mono-cycle).*

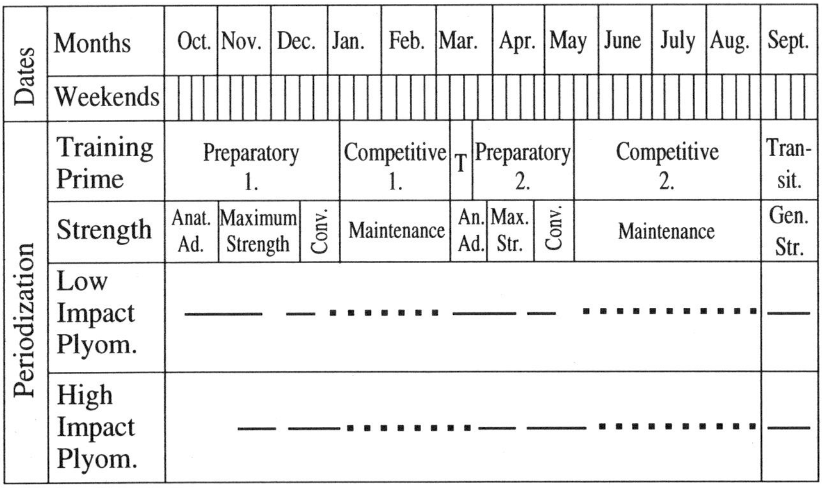

Figure 30 — Annual plan (bi-cycle)

	Months	Oct.	Nov.	Dec.	Jan.	Feb.	Mar.	Apr.	May	June	July	Aug.	Sept.
Dates	Weekends	‖‖‖‖	‖‖‖	‖‖‖	‖‖‖	‖‖‖	‖‖‖	‖‖	‖‖	‖‖‖	‖‖‖	‖‖	‖‖
Periodization	Training Prime	Preparatory 1.			Competitive 1.		T	Preparatory 2.		Competitive 2.			Tran-sit.
	Strength	Anat. Ad.	Maximum Strength	Conv.	Maintenance		An. Ad.	Max. Str.	Conv.	Maintenance			Gen. Str.
	Low Impact Plyom.												
	High Impact Plyom.												

Figure 30. *An example of an annual plan with only two peaks (bi-cycle).*

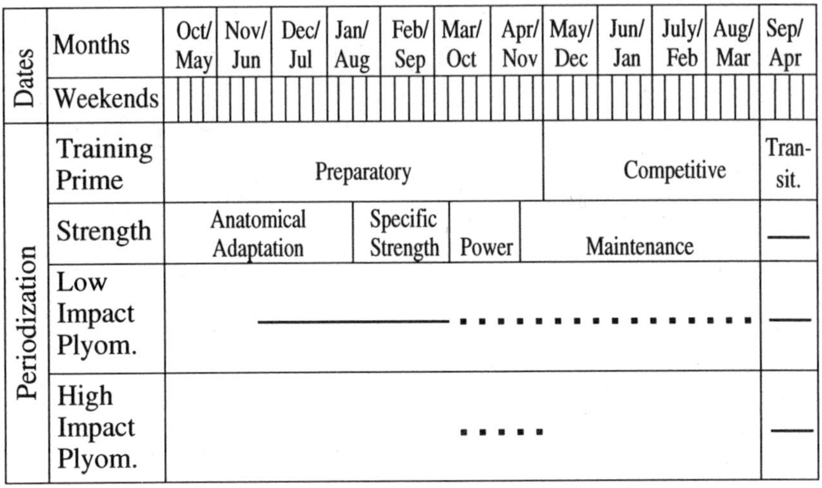

	Months	Oct/ May	Nov/ Jun	Dec/ Jul	Jan/ Aug	Feb/ Sep	Mar/ Oct	Apr/ Nov	May/ Dec	Jun/ Jan	July/ Feb	Aug/ Mar	Sep/ Apr
Dates	Weekends												
Periodization	Training Prime	Preparatory							Competitive				Tran-sit.
	Strength	Anatomical Adaptation				Specific Strength	Power		Maintenance				—
	Low Impact Plyom.	——————————— · · · · · · · · · · · · · · ·											—
	High Impact Plyom.	· · · · ·											—

Figure 31. An example of periodization of strength training for junior athletes.

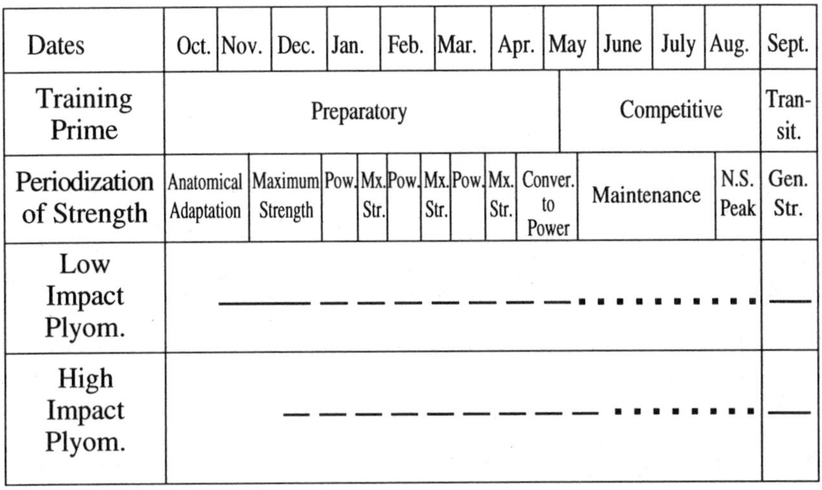

Dates	Oct.	Nov.	Dec.	Jan.	Feb.	Mar.	Apr.	May	June	July	Aug.	Sept.
Training Prime	Preparatory							Competitive				Tran-sit.
Periodization of Strength	Anatomical Adaptation	Maximum Strength	Pow.	Mx. Str.	Pow.	Mx. Str.	Pow.	Mx. Str.	Conver. to Power	Maintenance		N.S. Peak	Gen. Str.
Low Impact Plyom.	——— — — — — — —· · · · · · · · ·											—
High Impact Plyom.	— — — — — — — · · · · · · ·											—

Figure 32. The periodization of strength and plyometric training for an international class athlete.

Periodization

66

The periodization of strength training shown in Figure 31 is drastically different from the one designed for advanced athletes. In order to adapt anatomically to the strain of plyometric training, this phase is very long (early October to mid January, or early May to mid-August). Throughout this phase the load is low, 40-60%, and increased very slowly and progressively.

Instead of a maximum strength phase, which certainly would challenge an unprepared young body, it is planned as a specific strength phase. This implies that exercises are selected to be specific to the needs of the sport, and addressed to the prime movers (the muscles performing the technical movement). However the load is still low, 50-70% of maximum. The power phase, replacing the conversion phase, is designed to use principally medicine balls, light implements, which allows the athlete to perform a fast contraction over a short period of time. This is followed by a maintenance phase of a combination of specific strength and power.

As far as plyometric training is concerned, a December to early March or June to early October program of low impact plyometrics, is followed by high impact exercises, but only employing intensity level #3. This is planned only for the "power" phase. Low impact exercises are then maintained during the competitive phase.

Figure 32 attempts to present an example of the periodization of strength and plyometric training for an international class athlete (assumed to be involved in strength training for 6-8 years). It is also assumed that gains in maximum strength have leveled off, and therefore some innovations are necessary to break the usual pattern of periodization of strength training.

When adaptation of strength has reached a plateau which cannot be surpassed through traditional maximum strength methods, some new element of greater stimulation usually has to be tried. The innovation illustrated in Figure 32, represents the alternation of maximum strength phases of three weeks with two weeks of power training. By using strength training with a load of 50-70% of maximum--which permits a much faster muscle contraction--as well as light equipment (i.e. medicine balls) and high impact plyometric exercises, the athlete will be presented with new and powerful stimuli, which will eventually result in overcoming the present ceiling of adaptation and the attainment of superior levels of maximum strength and power.

As for the plyometric exercises, they follow the previously explained alternation of low with high impact exercises. As in the other examples (Figures 28 - 30), plyometrics are employed throughout the competitive phase to add to the maintenance of power, and/or power-endurance. The one exception, however, is the last two weeks before the main competition of the year, usually placed at the end of the competitive phase. During these two weeks, high impact plyometrics (intensity level #1-3) are used to stimulate a high level of neural activation, which can facilitate a "peaking" of the nervous system. This neurological peaking (Schmidtbleicher, 1984) can follow the simple model of Figure 33.

Week 1	Week 2	
Plyometrics (Activate the nervous system)	Unloading	Game/Race

Figure 33. The model of nervous system peaking.

During the first 10 days of the last two weeks prior to the main competition of the year, additional nervous system activation is induced by high impact plyometrics. The last 3-4 days before the game/race, unloading is scheduled, where the dominant elements of training are of a light technical/tactical nature. By applying this peaking strategy the athlete overcompensates for the competition, as well as activating the nervous system in order to produce the highest level of performance of the year.

Long-Term Planning
Long-term planning is one of the characteristics and requirements of modern training. A well-organized and planned training program over a long period of time greatly increases the efficiency of preparation for future major competitions. In addition, it encourages a rational

utilization of means and methods of training and facilitates a concrete, specific assessment of the athlete's progress. Organizing plans of 8-12 years duration should be a common approach for everyone who wants to be successful in the long term. Such an approach will increase the probability of reaching superior results at the age of athletic maturity.

During the athlete's competitive life the dynamics of physical and psychological development alter quite frequently. The motor and physiological functions reach an optimal level between the age of 20 and 30 years for men, and about 3-5 years earlier for women. However, it may not be inferred from this that the above ages are necessarily optimal for peak performance in all sports. For instance, optimal performance in sports requiring maximum speed is achieved by athletes around the age of 20-26 years. Similarly, activities requiring a great deal of strength and endurance are performed optimally by athletes approaching the age of 25 years and quite often even a little older. On the other hand, for sports in which success depends on the mastery of movement which can be acquired at an early age, the optimal age is significantly lower (figure skating at 16-20 years, gymnastics at the age of 14-16 years for girls and 18-24 years for boys).

The periodization of long-term training is suggested in Figure 34. Although variations to the model depend on the specifics of the sport and the dynamics of the individual athlete's development, programs for children can first be divided into two main phases.

From the age of 6-14 years a generalized program is suggested, where most kinds of activities, from running to climbing, from swimming to playing ball, are all desirable and contribute to the motor development of the future athlete. Although a lot of time is spent on technical development in the chosen sport, the limiting factor of performance for this age is technique, i.e. the proficiency of performing effectively the principal skills of the sport. However, this reality should not cause the coach to panic. Since technical perfection can be reached in some 8-12 years of practice, it would be quite inappropriate to expect technical miracles after 2-4 years of activity. Therefore, considering the scope of a long-term goal in training, namely that superior and effective performance has to be reached at maturity, during the "generalized" program the coach would be well-advised to invest the time in putting in place a good physical foundation for competition.

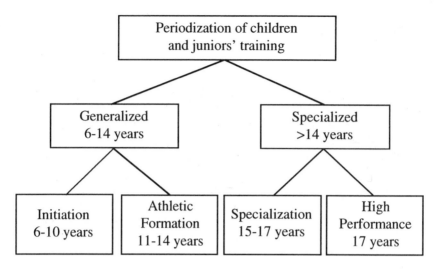

Figure 34. The periodization of long-term athletic development. (The proposed phases consider the normal dynamics of maturation.)

Over the age of 14 years, athletes can start the specialized program. This means that the coach will become increasingly concerned with the athlete's technical and tactical training, at the same time directing the program towards specific physical training. With some individual variations and differences between the needs of some sports, the limiting factor for this phase is still physical training.

An appropriate explanation for this is that as the athlete's technique improves and approaches perfection, the principal and most visible differences between leading competitors is not technique, but rather physical training, the very capacity which makes the athlete faster, stronger, and capable of enduring fatigue for a longer period of time.

Each of these two main branches is divided into two shorter and more specific training phases: the Generalized phase is divided into Initiation (6-10 years) and Athletic Formation (11-14 years). Having passed through these two "all-round" training phases, the coach can start specific training (Specialization, 15-17 years), leading progressively to the beginning of the High Performance training phase (for the 17 year olds and over).

A simple yet comprehensive presentation of each of these four phases is offered below, where both the objectives and training techniques ("Training Methods") are presented.

The Initiation Phase (6-10 years)
Training Objectives:
1. Multilateral (overall) physical and technical training, by exposing the child to various movements and technical skills.
2. Develop a harmonious body structure as well as correct body posture.
3. Develop coordination, balance, flexibility, and perception of various movements.
4. Develop aerobic endurance without exposing the child to stressful activities.
5. Develop concentration, imagination, discipline, and willpower to complete a training task.
6. Take part in only a few competitions and avoid stressing the role of victory. Competitions can also be fun.
7. The volume of training hours per year should be between 100-300 (for some sports even higher).

Training Methods:
1. Initiation in the technique of running, and simple jumping and throwing (e.g. baseball)
2. Develop and improve the skills of swimming, basic gymnastics, cycling, skating and skiing.
3. Learn to handle the ball in various team sports, through playing games with simplified rules.
4. Exercises with and on various apparatus.

The Athletic Formation Phase (11-14 years)
Training Objectives:
1. Develop the child's working capacity through general and multilateral (all-round) physical preparation.
2. Improve flexibility, coordination, aerobic endurance, thereby building the basis for speed and strength development.
3. Stress the acquisition of good technique, especially in the sport of future specialization.
4. Develop the perception of correct technical performance.
5. Based on specific tests towards the end of this phase, athletes should be directed to participate in sports in which they are seen to have ability.
6. Participate in competitions selected in accordance with individual potential.

71

7. Improve the concentration span, enthusiasm for the sport, determination, and will power.
8. Improve individual and team tactics, with special emphasis on offense.
9. Increase the volume of training hours per year to 300-400.

Training Methods:
1. Exercises for the improvement of general and specific training.
2. Exercises for the improvement of flexibility, coordination.
3. Exercises for the development of aerobic endurance, irrespective of the specifics of the sport.
4. Exercises against resistance (body weight and light apparatus).
5. Participation in competitions with events from the chosen and related sports (e.g. poliathlon, or a combination of several events).
6. Avoid participation in events requiring anaerobic endurance (e.g. 200m, 400m, 600m run) and triple jump because training for such events is too taxing for an immature body.

The Phase of Specialization (15-17 years)
Training Objectives:
1. In this the most important phase in training junior athletes, the main task is based on finding objective and subjective methods of directing the athlete to a sport/event in which to specialize.
2. Improve the motor abilities which are dominant in the selected sport/event.
3. A harmonious development of all bodily functions with great emphasis placed on those which ensure a high level of physical efficiency (i.e. endurance).
4. Increase both the volume and intensity of training but still without reaching a state of complete exhaustion.
5. Perfect technique for the selected sport/event.
6. Perfect individual tactics and improve team tactics.
7. Develop psychological abilities in accordance with the specifics of the selected sport.
8. Increase the volume of hours of training to 500-600 per year.

Training Methods:
1. Specific exercises are given priority, but exercises with related effects or multilateral development, are still an important component of training.

2. Exercises for improving flexibility and coordination.
3. Exercises for improving aerobic endurance should be emphasized, while those intended to develop anaerobic endurance should now be introduced progressively.
4. Exercises for improving muscular endurance and power (load up to 80% of maximum).
5. Participation in competitions in the specialized sport/event without totally excluding related sports.

The Phase of High Performance (>17 years)
Training Objectives:
1. Achieve highest performance in the specialized sport/event.
2. Perfect the specific motor abilities which would represent the foundation of accomplishing high performance.
3. Stress volume and/or intensity of training in accordance with the needs and characteristics of the sport.
4. Perfect and master both technique and tactics according to the specifics of the sport.
5. Perfect psychological qualities, especially initiative, self control and coping with stress and frustration in both training and competition.
6. Improve athlete's theoretical knowledge of training.
7. Increase progressively the annual volume of training from 600 to 800 hours. As the athlete approaches international standards the volume of hours of training could go to 1000 or even higher.

Training Methods
1. Exercises emphasizing specificity are dominant (80%), while those for all-round development (20%) are included especially during the preparatory and pre-competitive phase.
2. Exercises to perfect the dominant motor abilities.
3. Exercises to perfect and master technical elements and skills.
4. Specific tactical drills to perfect tactical preparation. Such drills should also have a built-in physical component.
5. Relaxation training intended to increase motivation and facilitate the rate of recovery.

An important component of long-term planning is also the need to establish a comprehensive list of plyometric exercises and then to compile a progression, showing how these types of exercises will be applied over a long period. Although it is to be expected that some changes will be made over the years, the coach is strongly advised to follow the proposed progression as faithfully as possible.

An example of such a list of exercises and their progression is illustrated in Figure 35. At the top of the list is the age range of the athletes, followed by the periodization of long-term planning and the four phases discussed above.

On the left hand side is a progression of several kinds of plyometric exercises. It is important to note that they are divided into five groups, each of them representing a level of intensity as discussed in chapter 6. These intensities start with the lowest (#5), and for each level there are several groups of suggested exercises. For the earliest age group, less strenuous exercise is suggested. As the young athlete matures and develops better anatomical adaptation, exercises become progressively more challenging. However, it is quite clear that by the time an athlete is exposed to "hops and steps" typical of the triple jump, he or she already has 7-8 years experience.

The model suggested by Figure 35 could be altered by the coach in order to accommodate the specific needs of each sport. Decisions regarding at what age to start training, and in particular, certain simple plyometric exercises, have to be based on the rate of maturation and the age at which superior performance is achieved in that particular sport. Some examples will demonstrate that high performance is not achieved at the same age in all sports, e.g. track and field: 20-25 years; basketball: 23-28 years; boxing: 23-30 years; diving: 18-23 years; women's gymnastics: 14-18 years; wrestling: 24-28 years, etc.

In order to compile the chart, the coach could consider as a general guideline that to reach superior performance (national level and up), an athlete requires some eight years of training. Of similar importance is the fact that, under normal conditions, an athlete with a good background, who has not been burned-out during the initiation and athletic formation phases, can continue to be successful at that high level for 6-10 years.

Considering the above guidelines, the coach should decide when to start training, as well as the distribution of plyometric exercises. Figure 35 can be used as a general guide for progression.

As far as possible, the coach should follow this progression, in order to avoid strain and to allow the athlete to progressively adapt to different exercises specific to the sport, as well as to plyometric exercises. The instructor/coach should be very disciplined in following the established

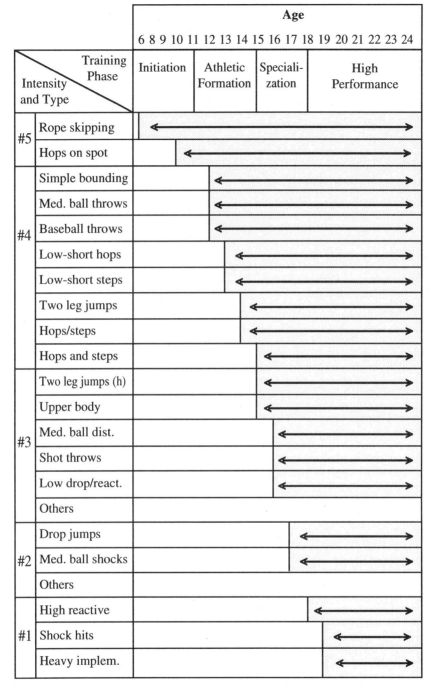

Figure 35.   Long-term planning: progression of plyometric exercises.

progression and should resist the temptation to show everything he or she knows in the first year(s)! This is the only way to produce an injury-free athlete.

The list of exercises incorporated in the chart can be quite large. However, it does not mean that all the exercises will be performed throughout the athlete's life. On the contrary! Take for instance the first exercise listed in Figure 35. This exercise could be a major component of the training program in the first few years, and employed only during the warm-up the following years.

Throughout the long-term plan, exercises must be chosen very selectively, based on the needs of the sport, the athlete's progress, as well as the particular phase of training of the annual plan. For a good selection of exercises, the reader is invited to consult the chapter on plyometric exercises.

PLYOMETRIC EXERCISES

Introduction

For the sake of convenience and in order to follow the progression illustrated by Figure 35 all the plyometric exercises are presented as per type of intensity: from intensity 5 to 1. However, since the exercises suggested for one category of athletes, for example intensity 3, are not present in intensity 2, it does not mean that they are excluded from training. On the contrary, the best exercises could be used by more advanced athletes as well.

For each category of intensity, exercises are presented in the following order:
·Single leg take-off exercises
·Double leg take-off
·Drop/reactive jumps, "shock" training.
·Upper-body exercises
·Relays and simple games

In each category, exercises may be divided into other classifications. However, before attempting to refer to each group of exercises separately, it is important to refer to some basic technical elements critical for correct execution.

Posture. While performing plyometric exercises, especially those over apparatus, the head has to be kept vertical with the chin up. This small postural detail is critical for two reasons:

1. The performer will be able to see around him, thereby eliminating the possibility of injuries caused by stepping or falling on balls, or on other apparatus in the gym.

2. If the chin is dropped while performing various hops or jumps over apparatus, it will start a slight forward rotation of the head and upper body, which may result in loss of body control and balance, and cause the athlete to fall to the floor or off onto a piece of apparatus. This may not cause an injury, but would certainly provide an unpleasant experience.

While performing plyometrics the upper body should always be kept vertical, and relaxed. The arms are either swung upward together in order to elevate the centre of gravity, or swung one at a time in coordination with the leg movements. In this way the arms will always counterbalance and thereby compensate the leg actions, resulting in well-coordinated movements.

An exercise in which the athlete travels over the ground in a single leg movement pattern is commonly known as a "bounding" exercise.

When the take-off (the propulsive force) is exerted by one foot and the landing is on the same one, the action is defined as a "hop". Following the take-off, the heel is tucked against the buttocks, followed by a rapid forward projection of the thigh towards the landing spot. The landing is very active, the athlete pulls through very rapidly, initiating another bound as soon as possible.

Landing in plyometric exercises is also a critical element. For most of the bounding exercises such as hops and steps, the landing is flat-footed, promptly followed by a rolling forward onto the toes and then the take-off (Figure 36).

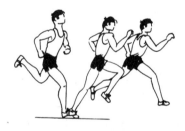

Figure 36.   The technique of landing for bounding exercises. Note the
             arm action at the moment of take-off.

A different landing technique is employed for reactive jumps. To facilitate a quick reaction, a dynamic stretching-shortening cycle, the landing for reactive jumps is performed on the ball of the foot, maintaining a locked ankle (Figure 37).

Figure 37. For reactive jumps, the landing is performed on the ball of the foot, and with the ankle locked.

If the landing is made on the other foot the action is defined as a "step" (or "leap"). The landing is active, followed by a rapid take-off accompanied by either a single or a double arm action (Figure 38).

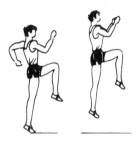

Figure 38. An example of a single or double arm action used for the take-off for "stepping".

While bounding may consist of single or multiple jumps, in a rhythmic coordination of leg and arm actions, the latter activities may be arranged in various combinations of left (L) and right (R) foot: L-L-R-R-L-R-L-L-R-R-etc.

Often during bounding, the conversion of horizontal velocity can be made into vertical lifts, or, in the vast majority of cases, into a flat and rhythmical forward action, where speed-reaction is the aim.

PLYOMETRIC EXERCISES FOR INTENSITY 5

Rope Skipping

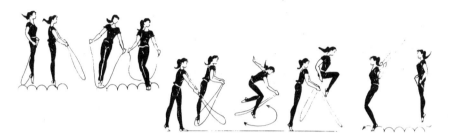

Figure 39. Rope Skipping.
Using single, alternate, or double leg action, where the emphasis is on continuous rebounding off the ground, rope skipping represents one of the most commonly used plyometric exercises. Variations include: circling underneath, forwards, backwards, sideways or in different geometrical shapes.

Single Leg Take-Off Exercises

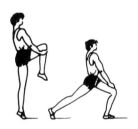

Figure 40. Lunge Steps.
Starting Position (SP) Standing, Movement (M): drive the knee upward followed by a long stride forward, immediately rebound and continue alternating with each leg.

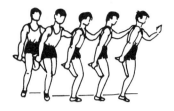 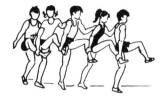

Figure 41   *Sequential Hops.*
SP: Hold one leg or grip the ankle of another athlete. M:
Sequential hops: forward, backward, sideways. While the
hops could be performed individually, an Indian file could
involve more athletes.

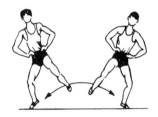

Figure 42   *Sideways Skips.*
SP: Standing, feet apart. M: Active take-off on left leg,
driving the right leg (thigh to horizontal) to the opposite
side. Land, quickly absorb the shock, and immediately
perform similar movements in opposite direction.

Simple Bounding Exercises With/Over Benches

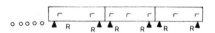

Figure 43   *Step on Bench.*

Place 2-4 gym benches end-to-end. SP: Athletes line up at the end. One by one the athletes step with the left leg on the top of the bench, extend the left leg actively, land on the right leg on the floor beside the bench, continuing the same to the end of the benches.

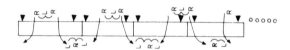

Figure 44   *Variation: -step on the top, then over, back on the top, over, etc.*
-step directly over the bench.

NOTE: When stepping on the bench, have the athletes place the foot exactly in the middle. Stepping on it, close to the edge, may roll the bench over and is potentially dangerous.

Exercises on Stairs

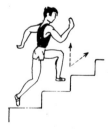

Figure 45   *Running Uphill and Downhill.*

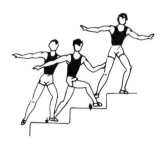

Figure 46   *Running Sideways, Crossing Legs Over.*

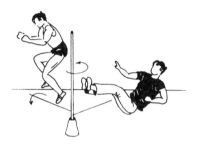

Figure 47   *Gladiator's Roulette.*
    Build a roulette (Figure 47) with two arms. As the vertical shaft is rotating, two athletes can either constantly jump over the arms, or, as in Figure 47, as one jumps the other lifts the legs to involve the abdominal muscles.

PLYOMETRIC EXERCISES FOR INTENSITY 4

Exercises on Stairs

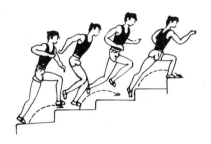

Figure 48   Running Up Two Stairs.

NOTE: Several variations of this exercise, and combinations are possible such as:
· alternate running over 1 and 2 stairs
· a hop over 1 stair with pause leg followed by running over 2 stairs
· combine hops with 1 and 2 legs, over 1 or 2 stairs
· running over 3 stairs

Single Leg Take-Off Exercises

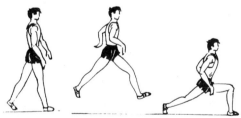

Figure 49   Scissors Splits.
SP as above, M as above, but the rebound is followed by a jump when the legs are switched quickly in midair. Look for maximal vertical height and an active take-off. Although the exercise is performed on the spot, the athlete should also try to go forward.

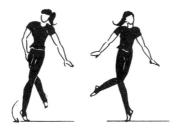

Figure 50 Side Scissors.
      SP: Standing, feet apart. M: Vertical jump, switching legs in midair, and land in starting position.

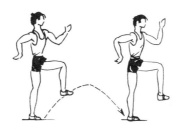

Figure 51 One Side Skipping.
      SP: Standing. M: Drive up the right leg and the left arm in coordination, take off and land on the same (right) leg. Alternate sequences on the right and left leg.

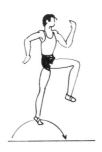

Figure 52 Two Side Skipping.
      SP: Standing. M: Take off on the left leg, driving the right leg up, thigh to horizontal, arms in coordination with legs,

and land on the left leg. Right leg is actively lowered on the ground, performing an active take-off, and driving up the left thigh. Continue the same, constantly alternating legs and arms.

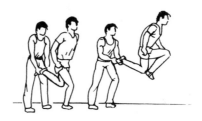

Figure 53 *Hopping On Spot.*
SP: Standing, left knee bent, ankle held by the coach or a partner. M: Take off on right leg, tucking the heel against the buttocks, knee being driven up towards the chest. Land, followed by an active rebound to continue for more hops. Perform series of hops, alternating legs.

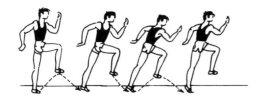

Figure 54 *Continuous Hops and Steps. Learn the skill and develop leg power by performing continuous hops and steps.*

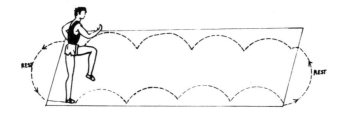

Figure 55 *Alternate Series of Hops and Steps on a Mat/Grass, with a rest interval at each end.*

OR:

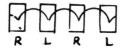

Figure 56

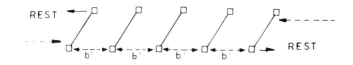

Figure 57 *Rhythm and Consistent Spacing.*
By using a series of marks, such as lines, ropes, or small circles, have the athletes keep a consistent cadence by landing on the marks.

NOTE: Throughout these drills ensure a flat-foot landing; absorb the shock by having the landing leg slightly bent and thus able to stretch into the next hop or step; stress the rhythm (cadence: Ta-Ta-Ta) of the series; keep chest high and relaxed; and drive into the next movement.

Informal Competition Between Athletes in activities such as:
- Three hops/or steps from standing start
- Penta-jumps (five steps/hops)
- Deca-jumps (ten steps/hops)
- The least number of hops in succession (R-R-L-L etc.) to cover a fixed distance.

Double Leg Take-Off Exercises
Jumps
Most exercises in this category of plyometric exercises are performed as a jump.

For the purpose of this book the characteristics of a jump are that the athlete takes off and lands on both feet simultaneously.

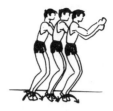

Figure 58   *Ricochets represents a low impact type of plyometrics in which the emphasis is on a rapid rate of take-offs and landings, minimizing the horizontal or vertical distance.*

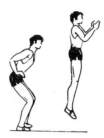

Figure 59   *Vertical Hops*
SP: Standing. M: Swing the arms upward and press actively against the ground for a vertical spring. Land, absorbing the shock, lowering the arms at hip level.

Bounding Exercises with Benches

Bounding Over Benches.
A series of possibilities are shown in Figures 60, 61, 62 and 63.

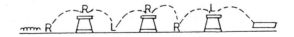

Figure 60

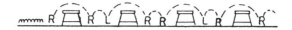

Figure 61

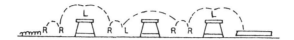

Figure 62

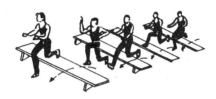

Figure 63

Figure 64   Note: *When the drill calls for stepping on the bench, an athlete could secure the bench by sitting on the end and holding it.*

Exercises with a Medicine Ball

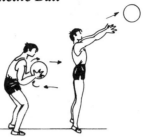

Figure 65   *Most medicine ball exercises are performed in a catch and throw manner. Throughout the throwing action the movement is performed progressively faster, maximum acceleration being achieved at the end. The catcher, on the other hand, anticipates the ball by extending the arms forward, to receive it. As the medicine ball is caught, the arms flex progressively, in order to absorb the shock. However, after absorbing the shock the momentum can be maintained, and by performing a semi-circular motion, the speed of the ball accelerates, culminating in another throw.*

For movements performed in positions other than "chest throws", the action might be slightly different, but the principle of accelerating throughout the range of motion is valid. After the catch, the speed of the ball is decelerated (absorbing the shock), changing the direction in preparation for the throw, and then accelerated for the final portion of throw.

Using a medicine ball can also create the "shock" reaction. Instead of absorbing the shock, one would catch the ball with the arms bent to a certain degree, usually around 110°-120°, without allowing any movement to occur. In this way a high tension in the muscles will be created, and the development of strength will be the normal outcome.

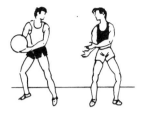

Figure 66   *Medicine Ball Twist-Throw.*

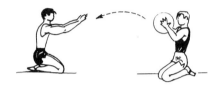

Figure 67   *Chest Throw.*

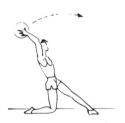

Figure 68   *Overhead Throw.*

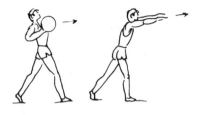

Figure 69   *Standing Chest Throw.*

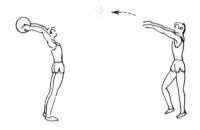

Figure 70   *Standing Overhead Throw.*

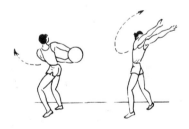

Figure 71   *Two-Hand Side Throw.*

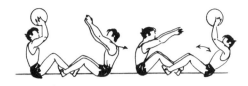

Figure 72   *Sit-Up Throw.*
SP: Partners sit on the floor, facing each other, with feet interlocked to secure good balance and support for the actions. One partner holds the ball above the head.
M: The ball is thrown towards the partner, who catches it, rocks backward and immediately changes the direction forward, releasing the ball towards his partner, for a maximal involvement of abdominal muscles.

Throws in Various Group Formations

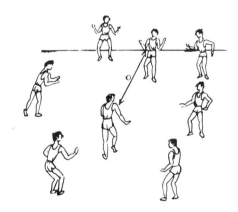

Figure 73   *All of the above suggested medicine ball throws could be performed in a "circle" (Figure 73), or in a "zigzag" formation (Figure 74). This could represent additional interest and variety in the daily routines.*

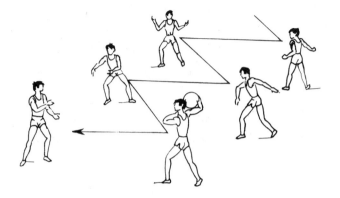

Figure 74

PLYOMETRIC EXERCISES FOR INTENSITY 3

Exercises on Stairs

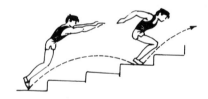

Figure 75 *Double-Leg Jumps on Steps, Over One, and Then Two .*

Single Leg Take-Off Exercises

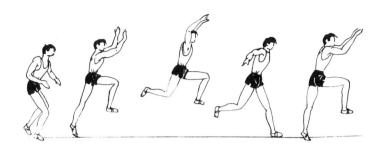

Figure 76   *Alternate Leg Bound.*
SP: standing, left foot slightly back. M: Push with the left leg against the ground, driving the right knee upward toward the chest, and forward, in order to gain distance. Land on right foot, and immediately rebound, driving the left knee upward-forward. Continue alternating take-off leg.

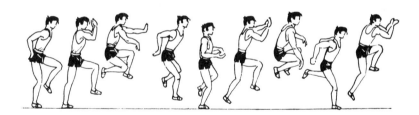

Figure 77   *Single Leg Hop.*
SP: Standing. M: Drive right leg up, and then reach forward to gain distance. Land on the same foot, continue the hops, while the left leg is held in stationary position throughout the exercise. Note that the arms are gathered together before landing, and swung upward-forward as the explosive take-off is performed.

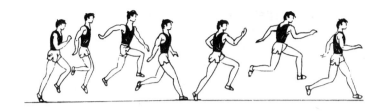

Figure 78 Standing Triple Jump.
SP: Standing, feet together. M: Drive one leg up and
forward for a controlled hop, land on same leg, drive the
opposite leg upward-forward for a controlled step, and
land on a mat/sandbox.

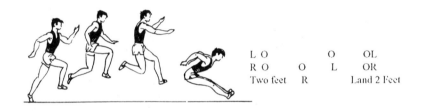

L O		O		OL
R O		O	L	OR
Two feet	R			Land 2 Feet

Figure 79 Figure 79 illustrates the same action by showing how the
right (R) and left (L) leg act in a standing triple jump.

Suggested Combination of Bounding Exercises using a Combination
of Hops, Steps, On, Off and Over Apparatus (walking or running).

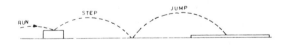

Figure 80

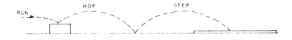

Figure 81

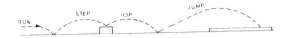

Figure 82

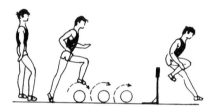

Figure 83

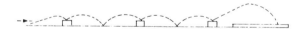

Figure 84

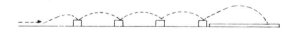

Figure 85

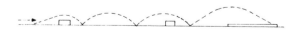

Figure 86

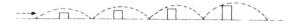

Figure 87

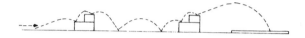

Figure 88

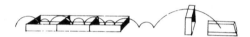

Figure 89

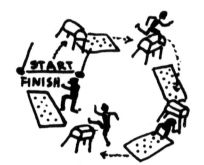

Figure 90

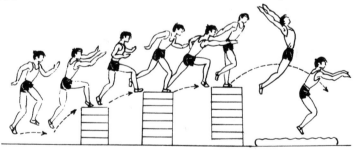

Figure 91

Double Leg Take-Off Exercises

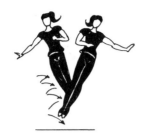

Figure 92   Slalom Jumps.
          *SP: Standing. M: Two-feet continuous diagonal jumps,
          progressing forward in slalom fashion.*

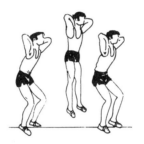

Figure 93   Squat Jumps.
          *SP: Standing, feet apart, hands behind the head. M: Active
          upward-forward movements. Land on toes, lower heels,
          and slightly bend the knees to absorb the shock, and repeat
          the sequence.*

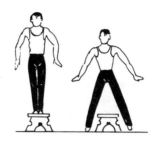

Figure 94   *Bench Jumps.*
> *SP: Standing on top of bench. M: Jump down, landing with one foot on either side of the bench. Swing arms upward, and immediately jump up, landing on the top (middle) of the bench, and repeat the action.*

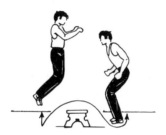

Figure 95   *Jump Over the Bench.*
> *SP: Standing, facing the bench. M: Jump over the bench, turn around, and immediately jump over again.*

Upper Body Exercises

These exercises are classified and presented according to the body part involved or the objects used. It should also be stated that some of them, especially the ballistic ones, involve most parts of the body, so the benefits are more comprehensive.

The progression in all the exercises, begins with the most simple ones, leading up to the "drop" or "shock" exercises, where high tension in the muscle is induced by the falling action of the body or machine. In exercises performed explosively, power is the end result, whereas "drop" exercises may result more in strength development. Since most figures are self-explanatory, description of movements will be minimal.

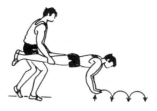

Figure 96   *Wheelbarrow.*
Whereas this exercise is normally "walking" on hands, for the purpose of plyometric training it is performed in small, forward hops.

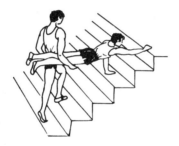

Figure 97   *Upstairs Wheelbarrow*
Note: Perform it at first by "walking" up, and then by "hopping" upstairs.

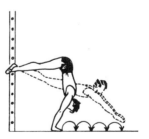

Figure 98   *Stall Bars Hops.*
SP: Feet up on a higher rung, both hands on the ground to reach an upside down position. M: for wards and backwards hops.

101

Exercises For Abdomen Muscles

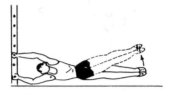

Figure 99   Side Lifts.

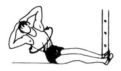

Figure 100   Trunk Twists.

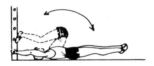

Figure 101   Overhead Lifts.

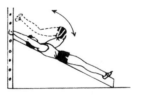

Figure 102   Inclined Overhead Lifts.

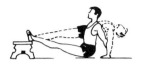

Figure 103   *Hip Thrusts.*
SP: Seated, heels resting on top of a bench, knees slightly bent, palms on the floor behind the hips, fingers pointing towards the bench. M: The hips are thrust upwards, and lowered onto the floor to continue the movement.

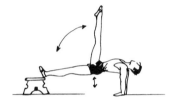

Figure 104   *Hip Thrusts Leg Lifts.*

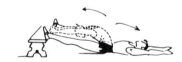

Figure 105   *Sit-Ups*

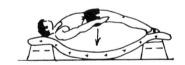

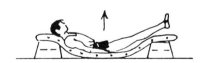

Figure 106   *Hammock Hip Thrusts.*

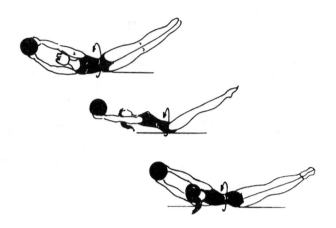

Figure 107　　*Abds Rolls.*
SP: The performer lies on the back, arms overhead holding a medicine ball. M: The hips are slightly flexed, the performer then rolls over onto the stomach, arching the back, then keeps rolling over hips to complete the rotation.
Note: Throughout these continuous rotations in both directions, avoid touching the floor with the legs, upper body and arms in order to better involve the back and abdominal muscles.

Trunk Extension Exercises

These often neglected trunk exercises strengthen and develop the low back and spine muscles (intervertebral ligaments and muscles). In order to qualify as plyometrics, these exercises have to be performed differently from the traditional ones. The difference lies in the fact that plyometrics have to be performed quickly and vigorously, especially the changing of direction from the rest or flexion position to extension. Some exercises could also be performed against the resistance provided by a partner, so the outcome would be a "shock" reaction, where the muscles are contracted instantly and more actively.

Note: Since trunk and hip extension exercises can result in injury, it is highly advisable that the coach strictly enforces the following rules:

1. Do not overextend - begin with a moderate range of motion.
2. Progress gradually to ensure the athlete has adapted to the work-load.
3. Only advanced athletes should perform these exercises.
4. The coach should be present throughout the session to observe and ensure that the above rules are strictly enforced.

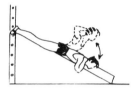

Figure 108.   *Trunk Thrusts*

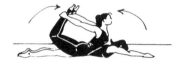

Figure 109   *Leg and Trunk Extensions.*

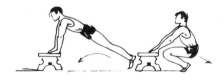

Figure 110   *Legs Thrusts.*

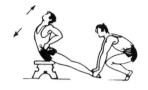

Figure 111   *Hip Extensions.*
SP: Performer rests his hips on a bench, hands behind
the neck, feet on the ground, ankles held by a partner.
M: The upper body is lowered slowly towards the
floor, then the direction changed quickly, by lifting the
trunk as high as possible.

Variation: As the trunk is lifted, the coach can block the
extension by placing the palms on the upper back, to
produce a "shock" reaction.

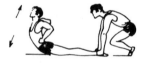

Figure 112   *Variation: The same exercise can be performed on the*
floor.

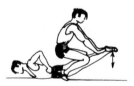

Figure 113   *Plyometric Leg Thrusts.*
SP: Performer lies on the stomach on the floor, the
partner seated near the ankles. M: Performer lifts the
legs as high as possible. As the legs approach the
highest point, the partner blocks the action by placing
the palms on the lower calves.

Ballistic Exercises

Substantial plyometric training benefits can be gained by performing exercises using a medicine ball, a shot from athletics and other similar objects. A very quick toss of an object involves the muscles of the body in a typical form of any plyometric exercises. In fact, since the force is performed against a light resistance in the shortest possible period of time, power of a most explosive type can be developed, so typical for the needs of the "conversion to power" phase (please refer to Chapter 7, and the Periodization of Strength).

Exercises With A Medicine Ball

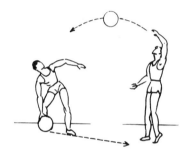

Figure 114   One-Arm Overhead Throw.

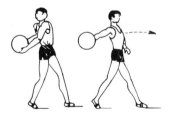

Figure 115   One-Arm Side Throw.

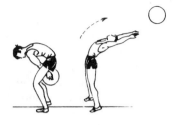

Figure 116   *Back Throw.*

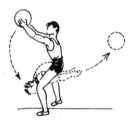

Figure 117   **Between the Legs Throw.**

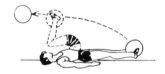

Figure 118   *Back Roll and Throw.*

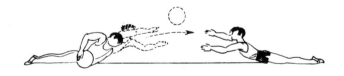

Figure 119   *Side Throw.*

108

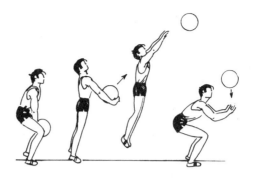

Figure 120   *Scoop Throw.*
SP: Assume a half-squat position, feet apart, arms
extended down between legs, holding the ball. M:
Extend legs in an active take-off while the arms swing
upward, releasing the ball vertically upwards. After
landing, catch the ball with both palms, return to a half
squat position, then repeat.

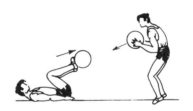

Figure 121   *Double Leg Kick.*
SP: Performer lays on his back, legs tucked to the
chest, while the partner stands in front of him 2-3m (7-
10ft) away, holding the ball. M: Ball is tossed towards
the balls of the feet of the performer. Before the ball
touches the feet, the performer kicks both legs, hitting
the ball vigorously towards the standing partner.

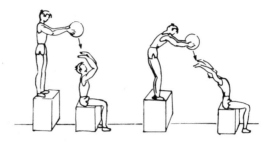

Figure 122   *Two Hand Hit.*
SP: Performer is seated on a bench (box), arms above head, palms up, elbows flexed. The partner stands on a higher box, holding the ball. M: Ball is released down towards the palms of performer. Just before the ball touches the palms, elbows are actively extended, hitting the ball upward.

Exercises With Light and Heavy Implements

A variety of plyometric exercises can be performed using baseballs, batons, 400-800gm (1-2 lb) bars, shots from track and field, or heavy bags.

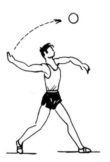

Figure 123   *Baseball Throw (for right-handed thrower).*
SP: Standing, left leg forward, right leg back, right arm, holding the ball, behind and slightly above the shoulder. M: Drive the left arm and shoulder side ways, drive the throwing arm over the shoulder and forward, culminating in a forward throw for distance.

Variations: Throw the ball with one step, three steps (as in the javelin throw), or perform the same with the opposite arm. Same throws could be performed with short sticks 20-40 cm (12-24 in.) long.

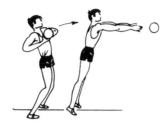

Figure 124   *Two-Arm Chest Shotput.*
SP: Standing, feet apart, shot held on both palms and fingers, in front of chest. M: Upper body is slightly arched, followed by upper body forward move, actively extending the arms in a forward throw.

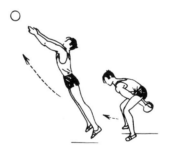

Figure 125   *Between Legs Forward Shot Throw.*
SP: Feet at shoulder width, shot held on both palms, facing the direction of the throw. M: Flex the hips, swing the arms back between the legs, flexing the knees as well. Swing the upper body and arms forward, extending the knees actively, and release the shot forward.

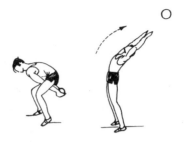

Figure 126   *Between Legs Backward Shot Throw.*

Variations: Both throws *(Figure 125 and 126)*   can be performed using heavy bells *(Figure 127)* of 5 kg (11 lb.), 7.5 kg (16 lb.), 10 kg (22 lb.), 15 kg (33 lb.) or heavier. To facilitate the throw, the performer lifts the weight by the handle on the bell.

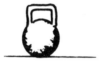

Figure 127   *Throwing Bell*

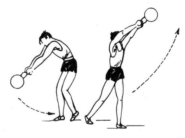

Figure 128   *Large Rotation Bell Throw.*
SP: Standing, feet apart, arms down, holding the bell.
M: Swing the upper body to the right, immediately change the swing to the left, accelerate as much as possible, ending with an active side throw.

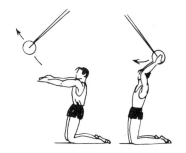

Figure 129   *Two-handed Overhead Toss.*

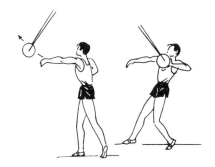

Figure 130   *One-Arm Put.*

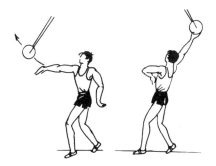

Figure 131   *One-arm Overhead Toss.*

113

Variation: - Perform same in the opposite direction.
               - Perform 1-2 large upper body rotations before
                 the throw.

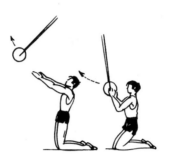

Figure 132   *Two-hand Swinging Shot/Bell Press.*
                 Implement: suspend a bell/shot on the ceiling. SP:
                 Kneeling, holding the implement in front of the chest.
                 M: Press the weight forward.

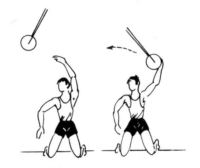

Figure 133   *One-Arm Side Toss.*

Note: Since the swinging of a heavy implement could be dangerous, it is highly advisable that the coach strictly enforces the following rules:
1) no other athletes should be in the radius of the swinging implement.
2) a stopping device for the implement should be secured (e.g. a hook).
3) after the throw, the athlete should move to the side, to be sure of avoiding being hit by the swinging implement.
4) only mature athletes should perform this and the following exercises.
5) the coach should be present throughout the session to observe and ensure that the above rules are strictly adhered to.

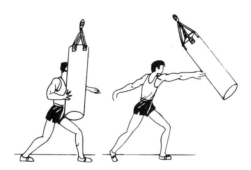

Figure 134   *Heavy Bag Thrust.*
SP: Take a semi-split position, half turned towards the bag, placing the palm of the performing arm on the bag. M: Swing the shoulder and actively push the bag away from the body. Stop the returning bag abruptly in order to create the "shock" reaction of the muscles involved.

Variations: - alternate arms
- push the bag sideways, arm extended, maximum upper body rotation
- standing behind the bag make a two-hand thrust, and stop the bag for "shock" reaction

Single Leg Take-Off Exercises

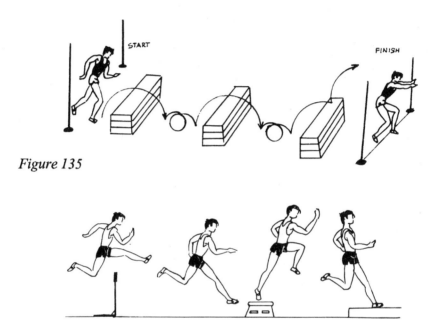

Figure 135

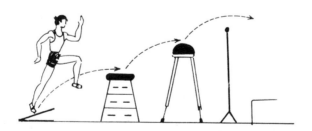

Figure 136

Figure 137

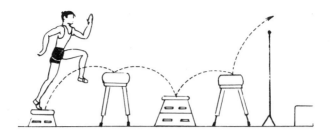

Figure 138

Double Leg Take-Off Exercises

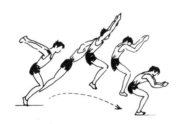

Figure 139 *Standing Long Jumps.*
SP: Standing, feet parallel and hip-width apart. M: Swing arms backward, bending knees and hips. Swing arms forward, performing an explosive upward-forward movement. In midair, pull the knees up to the body. Land by extending the legs forward, and bend knees to absorb the shock.

117

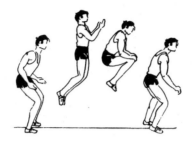

Figure 140 *Knee-Tuck Jumps.*
> *SP: Standing. M: Swing arms upward, actively pressing the feet against the ground for a vertical tuck jump. Land by flexing the knees to absorb shock.*

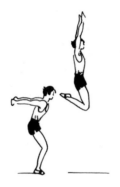

Figure 141 *Back Kicks.*
> *SP: Standing. M: Vertical jump bringing the heels to* buttocks.

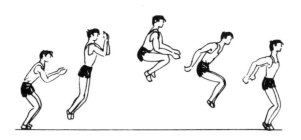

Figure 142 Double Speed Hop.
> SP: As above. M: Forward tuck jumps. Upon landing, jump quickly upward again to continue the sequence.

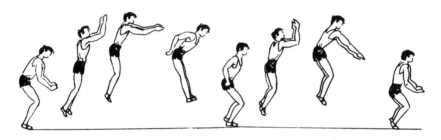

Figure 143 Standing Long Jumps.
> SP: As above. M: Forward double leg bound. Before landing bring legs forward, and upon landing resume starting position and quickly repeat.

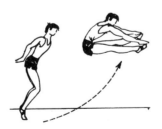

Figure 144 Frog Kicks.
> SP: Standing. M: Vertical jump, bringing the legs up and at the same time attempting to touch the toes. Bring legs quickly back down, under the body, land and spring up again to repeat the action.

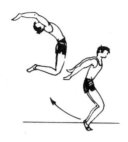

Figure 145 *Bow-Jumps.*
    *SP: Standing. M: Vertical jump, arching the body. Bring
legs quickly back down to absorb the shock.*
    Note: Start with individual jumps, aim to progress towards
performing a series of jumps.

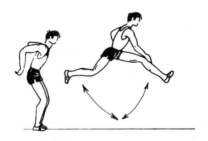

Figure 146 *Scissors Jumps.*
    *SP: Standing. M: Vertical jump, while in midair bring one
leg forward, the other backward, in a scissors-like movement. Repeat by alternating legs.*

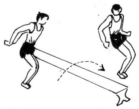

Figure 147 *Side Jumps Over the Bench.*
    *SP: Standing at the end of a bench (or series of benches,
end-to-end), one side facing the bench. M: Swing arms,*

jump over bench, land, make a small intermediate prepara-
tory jump on the spot, and jump over again. Continue the
actions.
NOTE: For advanced athletes, try to jump directly over,
without the preparatory jump.

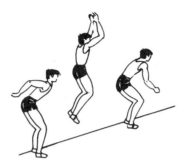

Figure 148 Incline Hops
NOTE: Performed as normal hops except that before
landing knees should be bent and brought forward more
than normal to clear the inclined slope.

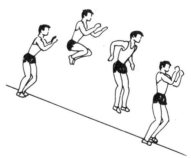

Figure 149   *Decline Hops*
Note: Due to the decline, pay maximum attention to
balance. Since the intent of this exercise is to empha
size speed of movement and high repetition rate, only
well-coordinated, or advanced athletes should use it.

Drop Jumps. Landing on the ground without yielding or jumping is an excellent method of developing strength. While reactive jumps and bounding exercises develop power, drop jumps are a form of exercise aimed at developing maximum strength.

Schmidtbleicher (1984) claimed that drop jumps, as compared to other forms of plyometric training and even strength training, create the greatest tension in the muscles. And the outcome is maximum strength development.

One element of progression is the height of the box. Verkhoshanski (1968) and other authors have tried experimental heights up to 3.20m (7.3 ft)! However, for training purposes an 2.6-3.6ft (.80-1.09m) is regarded as being adequate.

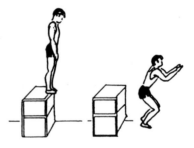

Figure 150   *Drop jump*
SP: Standing on the box, facing the direction of the drop-jump. M: Step down, landing on the balls of both feet without absorbing the shock by flexing knees or hips. Arms are used just to balance the body. After landing, relax legs, and immediately climb on the box again. Rest interval is taken only after performing a series of jumps.

Exercises For Upper Body

Exercises For Abdomen Muscles

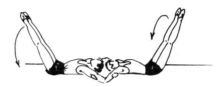

Figure 151   *Double Leg Side Lifts.*
SP: Two partners lie on their backs, heads close
together, gripping their hands for support and balance
during movement. M: Both lift up their legs, and then
bring them down in the opposite direction. After
reaching the floor they lift the legs in the opposite direc
tion, to continue the movement.
Variation. A "shock" reaction could be achieved if, at
a given signal, the movement of the legs is stopped
abruptly (before touching the ground) and the direction
of lift changed.

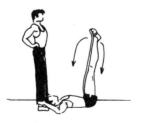

Figure 152   *Variation.*
SP: A partner stands, feet apart, while the performer
lies down, head near the partner's feet, hands gripping
the ankles. The performer lifts his legs as above.

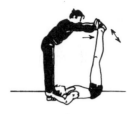

Figure 153   *"Abds Shocker".*
SP: As above. M: Performer lifts legs towards the chest of his partner. Before reaching the vertical position the ankles of performer are caught by the hands of the partner and recoiled downwards. These two opposing forces create a very high tension at the level of the abdominals. The performer brings the legs upwards again, and the action is repeated.

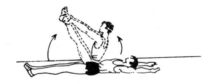

Figure 154   "V" Sits.

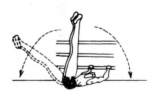

Figure 155   *Abds Rainbows.*
SP: The performer lies down, head near the lowest rung of a stall bar, hands gripping it. M: Legs are lifted and lowered on both sides.
Variation. A "shock" reaction is achieved if the lift of the legs is opposed by a partner.

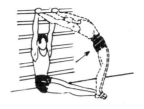

Figure 156   *Abds Arches.*
S.P. The performer is seated, back against the stall bars, arms above head, gripping the nearest rung. M: The hips are pressed actively upward arching the body (feet are on the ground, hands firmly gripping the rung). The hips are lowered to the starting position and the movement continued.

Exercises With A Medicine Ball

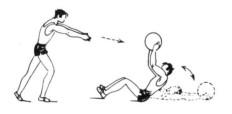

Figure 157   *Large Sit-Up Throw.*
SP: One partner stands, feet apart, holding the ball. The other is seated, feet apart, knees slightly flexed. M: Ball is carefully tossed towards the chest of the seated partner. As the ball is caught, the partner rocks towards the floor, then using the momentum of an upper body upward thrust, throws the ball back to the other partner.

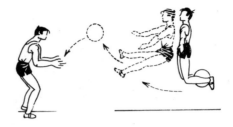

Figure 158   *Double Leg Forward Toss.*
SP: Two partners standing, 3 m (10 ft) apart, facing
each other. One of them grips a medicine ball between
the feet and toes (toes are also slightly under the ball).
M: The partner with the ball, performs a two foot take-
off. As he approaches the highest point, he slightly
arches the hips, bringing the feet backwards, as quickly
as possible, by forcefully contracting the abdominal
muscles, the legs are brought forward, releasing the
ball towards the chest of his partner who catches it,
and performs the same action.

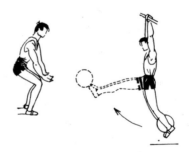

Figure 159   *Variation: Perform the same toss from hanging*
position.

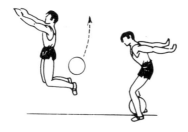

Figure 160   *Double Leg Backward Toss.*
Assume a similar position as in Figure 158 but the toss
is performed backwards and upwards.

PLYOMETRIC EXERCISES FOR INTENSITY 1

Reactive and Drop Jumps

Reactive jumps (often not very appropriately called "depth jumps") are jumps from an elevated position with an immediate rebound (or "reaction", therefore "reactive jumps").

Researchers such as Asmussen (1979) and Gollhofer, et al. (1987) compared the rebound, or reaction, with the temporary absorption and storage of kinetic energy by a rubber ball. When the ball hits the ground, after being dropped, it is deformed as it stores kinetic energy. As the ball retakes its original shape, energy will be released to bring the ball upward, to the height it was dropped from.

In reactive jumps, the kinetic energy of the athlete accelerates as a result of the pull of gravity, it is converted at ground contact into muscle tension--energy which is then utilized for the rebounding, or reactive phase (take-off).

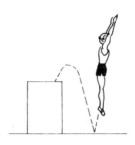

Figure 161   A standard reactive jump.

Landing in reactive and drop jumps is performed on the ball of the foot, with stiff ankles, and knees bent to an angle which allows amortization and a smooth and quick change into an upward drive. Exercises can be performed on one or two legs.

Although reactive jumps can be performed from various heights, an optimal elevation could be established through a simple test. Zanon (1977) recommends heights of 40 cm (16 in.) and 60 cm (24 in.). The heights of the reactive jumps are measured. For optimal training effect, the rebound height must exceed the previous elevation. The main factor in reactive jumps is the speed of the rebound, the transfer of energy from the eccentric to concentric phase. Ideally, the rebound is performed instantaneously, because any pause at the bottom of the jump results in a loss of transfer of energy, and so performance will be poor.

Single Leg Reactive Jumps

Of the multitude of heights, lengths, and movement types, a few examples are presented on the following page. Figure 162 illustrates a jump performed mostly vertically, while in Figure 163 the intent is also to advance as far forward as possible. Variations: take off with 180 or 360 degrees of rotation; jumps followed by alternate leg skips; jumps followed by a combination of bounds (Figure 164), and jumps followed by other reactive jumps using ropes, hurdles, cones, benches or boxes (Figure 165).

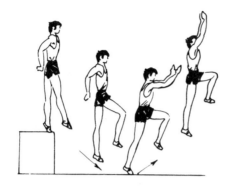

Figure 162

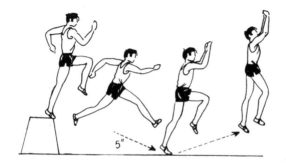

Figure 163

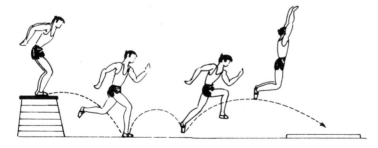

Figure 164

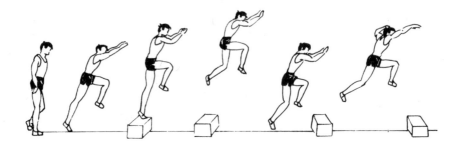

Figure 165   *Alternate and Single Leg Jumps*

Double Leg Reactive Jumps

Using boxes and hurdles the coach can create a multitude of combinations of jumps. Some are described below, the others are self-explanatory. A careful progression should be observed throughout. Progressions vary from the height of the box or hurdle, to whether the jump is a single one, or a series of jumps, and whether they are performed on and off the box, directly over the box in a series of reactive jumps, or with a stutter, small jump, followed by another jump over.

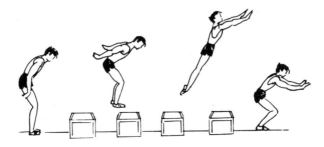

Figure 166   *Double Leg Box Bounds.*
SP: Standing, facing a row of boxes, spread out at equal distances, depending on the class of athlete. M: jump on and off the box, with maximum attention being paid to the immediate and explosive reactive jump performed on the floor. Constantly use arm swings for take-off or to balance the upper body.

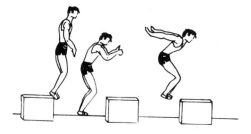

Figure 167   Reactive Box Jumps.
SP: Stand on the box, facing the row of boxes. M:
Land on the ground, explosive take-off to jump onto the
next box, using an active arm swing. 1-2 seconds
preparation for the next jump, and the activity is
continued over all the boxes.

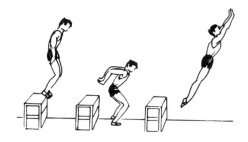

Figure 168   Reactive Jumps Over Boxes.
As above, except that this time the reactive jump is
performed directly over the boxes. For a better pro
gression, especially for the less skilled athletes, a
stutter jump is advisable.

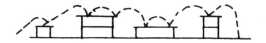

Figure 169

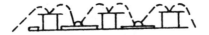

Figure 170

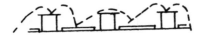

Figure 171

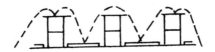

Figure 172

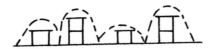

Figure 173

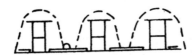

Figure 174

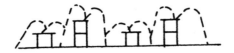

Figure 175

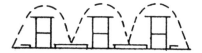

Figure 176

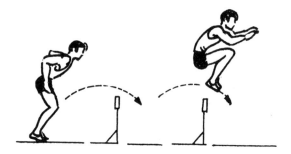

Figure 177   *Reactive Jumps Over Hurdles.*
SP: Standing, facing the hurdle(s). M: Swing arms
upward, active take-off to clear the hurdle, and upon
landing, spring immediately up and over again to clear
the next hurdle.

Note: These exercises can be performed at first with a
stutter jump, over one hurdle or more. Cones or cords
across two supports, can replace hurdles. The height to
clear and the space between hurdles is dependent on the
classification of athlete (Figures 177-179).

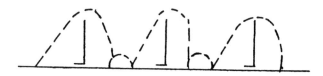

Figure 178

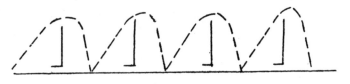

Figure 179

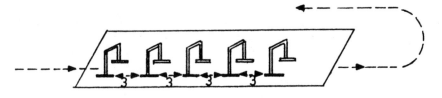

Figure 180   *A suggested arrangement for the hurdles*

Exercises For Upper Body

Exercises For Arms and Shoulders

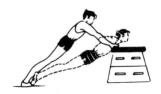

Figure 181   *Variations of Body Drops.*
Following each drop perform an explosive upwards
push (Figures 181, 182, 183, 184)

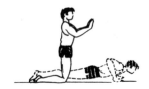

Figure 182

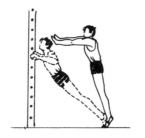

Figure 183

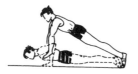

Figure 184

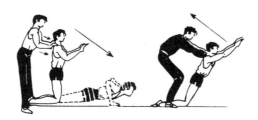

Figure 185   Catch and Drop Push-Ups.
SP. Performer kneels, the partner catches his upper
arms. M: Performer is allowed to drop onto the floor,
elbows flexed, and immediately makes a vigorous push
up towards the starting position.

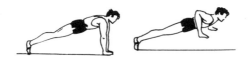

Figure 186   Plyometric Push-Ups

Exercises For Abdomen Muscles

From the numerous exercises available for the "abds" plyometrics, the selected ones are presented by Figures 187, 188 and 189. Please note that any exercises could be qualified as "shock" reaction, where the high tension generated in the muscles could be compared to the tension achieved by the leg extensors during "drop jumps". The athlete needs a partner to "oppose" the lifting action of a body segment. A simple example will illustrate the "shock" exercise: everybody knows the sit-up exercise; the very same exercise could qualify as a plyometric "shock" exercise if the partner stops the upward lift of the upper body at the midpoint.

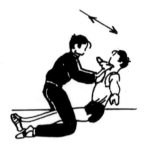

Figure 187   *Plyometric Sit-Ups.*
SP: Performer lies on the back, a partner kneels at the side, near the hips. M: Performer executes a sit-up and at the midpoint the partner stops the upper body lift, by placing a hand on the chest or shoulder of the performer.

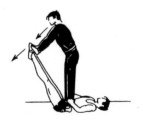

Figure 188   *Plyometric Leg Lifts.*
Similar actions are executed while the performer lifts the legs.

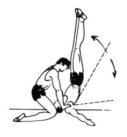

Figure 189   *Abds Kips.*

Simple Tumbling Plyometrics

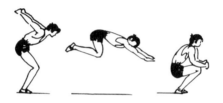

Figure 190   *Frog Leaps.*
SP: Low crouch, arms flexed in front of the chest. M:
Extend legs to perform a frog leap, land on hands first
and bring legs together, to return to starting position.

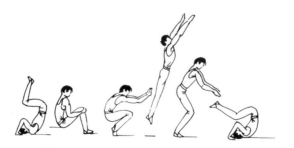

Figure 191   *Forward Roll and Verticle Jump.*
SP: As above. M: Tuck the head under and roll over
to a half-squat position, actively extend the legs to
perform a vertical jump. Land and repeat.

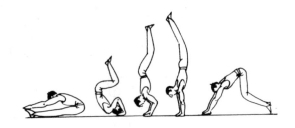

Figure 192   *Back Roll into Hand-stand.*
SP: Seated, chest above knees. M: The upper body is swung backwards, the shoulders rolled over, palms on ground, below shoulders. When approaching vertical, the arms are extended into a hand-stand. Legs are lowered into a low crouch, and then it is repeated.

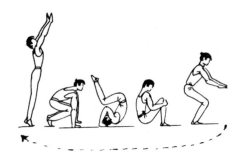

Figure 193   *Back Roll into a Vertical Jump.*
SP: Half-squat. M: The knees are fully flexed, and the performer rolls backwards into a full squat, performs an active vertical jump, lands, then repeats the movement.

Relays and Games

Plyometric exercises are both challenging and fun. The more combinations the coach can use, the more enjoyable they can be.

138

The development of power through plyometrics is possible not only through the groups of exercises suggested above, but also through the relatively relaxed training environment of relays and games.

During relays and games the athletes sprint, jump, carry and throw medicine balls, all of which are exercises which result in power gains. In addition the athletes enjoy doing them and at the same time can develop the team and competitive spirit. For all these reasons, relays and games are highly recommended.

In a well-structured training session, it is suggested that relays and games be employed at the end. Although the athletes may be tired, through the fun of relays and games they can still be challenged to go beyond the physical limitations imposed by fatigue.

Some relays and games are presented below. Use games from other books or try creating new games of your own. The athletes will welcome all the variety you can introduce into your sessions.

Relays

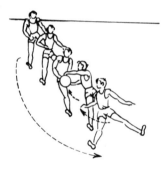

Figure 194   *Medicine Ball Side Pass.*
SP: Two equal teams, seated, feet apart, first player holds the ball. Distance between the players should be calculated so that the pass is performed comfortably. M: First player rotates to the right passing the ball to the next. This is continued as fast as possible to the end of the line. The last player stands up as quickly as possible, runs to the front, sits down and starts the series again. When the first player is at the end of the row, the relay is over. The winner is the team which finishes the relay first.
Variations: -pass the ball alternately to each side
        -pass the ball back over the head
        -hold the ball between feet, roll over, and pass the
        ball to the feet of the next player.

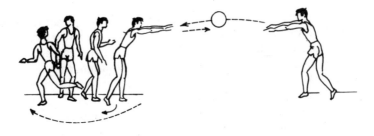

Figure 195   *Medicine Ball Chest Pass.*

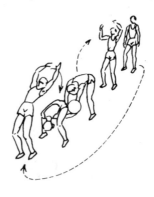

Figure 196   *Over-Under Bridge.*

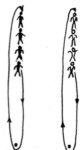

Figure 197   *File Relay.*
Carry the ball, roll it all the way, perform hops, steps, and double leg jumps, etc.

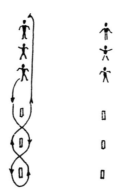

Figure 198   *Slalom Relay.*

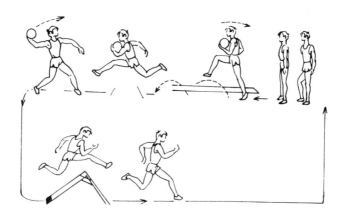

Figure 199   *Complex Relays.*
Note: Make sure that the distance between the apparatus is equal for both teams. Various apparatus or movements can be used.

Games

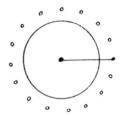

Figure 200

Rope Jump. A light ball (e.g. a volleyball) is placed in a net and attached to a rope. One athlete stays in the middle of the circle, and all the other athletes make a large circle, the radius of which is the length of the rope. The athlete from the centre rotates the ball continuously (ground level). As the ball approaches an athlete, he should jump to avoid being hit by the ball. Every time a player is hit, he is eliminated from the game. The winner is the last player left in the game. Note: The rope is progressively elevated at every third rotation, so that the athletes have to keep jumping higher. Make sure that the rope has the same height throughout its rotation.

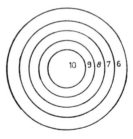

Figure 201

Baseball Dart Game.
Draw five circles on a wall. The inner circle is 30 cm (1 ft) in diameter, and subsequent circles to be drawn 15 cm (6 in.) apart. Values for each circle should be given as per Figure 201.
A line is drawn at 15 m (50 ft.), 22 m (75 ft.) and 30 m (100 ft.). Athletes have three throws from each distance, using overarm technique (like a javelin throw). Every time the ball hits an area, the athlete receives the specified score. The sum of all throws represents the final score for each athlete and all the athletes are ranked at the end of the game.

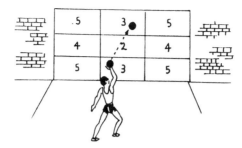

Figure 202   *Board Throws.*
Follow similar rules as above but throw at a board
where rectangles of 15 x 30cm (6 x 12 in.) are drawn
as per Figure 202.

Medicine Ball Speed Throws. Two rows of players, organized in pairs, facing each other, 5 m (15 ft) apart. Players from the right row have the ball. The aim of the game is to determine which pair can perform the most throws in 30 seconds (or 60, 90 and 120 seconds). The technique of throwing is to be determined by the coach.

Note: For "between the legs" forward/backward throws, the distance can be increased to 10-12 m (30-40 feet).

Medicine Ball "Volleyball" Game
Aim: To find which team is the faster to score 15 points in 2 of 3 games.
Rules: Two teams of 3 players are set in each court. The rules from volleyball will be followed, with the exception that the courts are smaller 3 x 3 m(10 x 10 ft) and instead of serving, the ball is thrown over the net into the opposite court.
Net: The highest point of the net (rope, band, etc.) will be set at the average shoulder height of the players.
Referee: The coach or a player.

Note: The court can be marked by tape, or a small but visible object in each corner. DO NOT use balls as markers, as they can cause injuries if a player steps on one. The duration of a set could also be limited by time, e.g. 3 sets of 5 minutes.

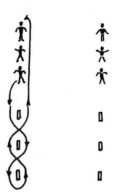

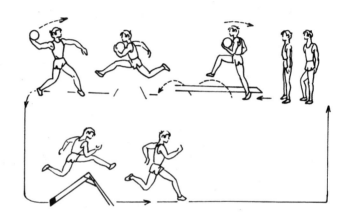

Figure 198.   *Slalom Relay.*

Figure 199.   *Complex Relays.*
                 Note: Make sure that the distance between the
                 apparatus is equal for both teams. Various apparatus
                 or movements can be used.

Games

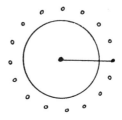

Figure 200.   *Rope Jump. A light ball (e.g. a volleyball) is placed in a net and attached to a rope. One athlete stays in the middle of the circle, and all the other athletes make a large circle, the radius of which is the length of the rope. The athlete from the centre rotates the ball c ontinuously (ground level). As the ball approaches an athlete, he should jump to avoid being hit by the ball. Every time a player is hit, he is eliminated from the game. The winner is the last player left in the game.* Note: The rope is progressively elevated at every third rotation, so that the athletes have to keep jumping higher. Make sure that the rope has the same height throughout its rotation.

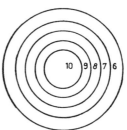

Figure 201.   *Baseball Dart Game.*
Draw five circles on a wall. The inner circle is 30 cm (1 ft) in diameter, and subsequent circles to be drawn 15 cm (6 in.) apart. Values for each circle should be given as per Figure 201.

    A line is drawn at 15 m (50 ft.), 22 m (75 ft.) and 30 m (100 ft.). Athletes have three throws from each distance, using overarm technique (like a javelin throw). Every time the ball hits an area, the athlete receives the specified score. The sum of all throws represents the final score for each athlete and all the athletes are ranked at the end of the game.

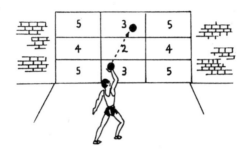

Figure 202.   *Board Throws.*
Follow similar rules as above but throw at a board
where rectangles of 15 x 30cm (6 x 12 in.) are drawn
as per Figure 202.

Medicine Ball Speed Throws. Two rows of players, organized in pairs, facing each other, 5 m (15 ft) apart. Players from the right row have the ball. The aim of the game is to determine which pair can perform the most throws in 30 seconds (or 60, 90 and 120 seconds). The technique of throwing is to be determined by the coach.

Note: For "between the legs" forward/backward throws, the distance can be increased to 10-12 m (30-40 feet).

Medicine Ball "Volleyball" Game
Aim: To find which team is the faster to score 15 points in 2 of 3
    games.
Rules: Two teams of 3 players are set in each court. The rules from
    volleyball will be followed, with the exception that the courts are
    smaller 3 x 3 m(10 x 10 ft) and instead of serving, the ball is thrown
    over the net into the opposite court.
Net: The highest point of the net (rope, band, etc.) will be set at the
    average shoulder height of the players.
Referee: The coach or a player.

Note: The court can be marked by tape, or a small but visible object in each corner. DO NOT use balls as markers, as they can cause injuries if a player steps on one. The duration of a set could also be limited by time, e.g. 3 sets of 5 minutes.

TESTING

Testing power normally refers to two types of capacity: to project an object (i.e. a medicine ball), and to project one's body (i.e. standing long jump).

In most cases such tests are relatively simple, consisting of exercises used during training sessions. However, sometimes the performers, especially beginners, should be taught a particular skill and given adequate practice time.

One of the main advantages of the following power tests is that they are relatively easy to administer, employ simple equipment, and produce meaningful results. These results can then be recorded and referred to throughout the annual plan, as a measure of the athletes' improvement in power.

The force of acceleration is the main stimulus for power training, so this is the quality to be tested. Test items should be selected in such a way that they involve maximal or near maximal contraction performed against the force of gravity or against resistance in a minimum period of time. "What is actually measured then, is the distance through which the body or an object is propelled through space as a result of the power performance" (Gledhill, 1987).

In order to have consistency throughout the year(s), the same test items, and in the case of implements, the same weight, should be utilized.

Upper Body Tests

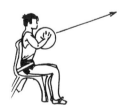

Figure 203. Medicine Ball Chest Throw. The ball is close to the chest with both hands, elbows flexed

Equipment and Marking: Medicine ball 4-7 kg (9, 12 or 15 lb.); a throwing area where longer throws could be performed and imme diately measured.

Starting Position: Seated, legs flat on the floor, hips or chest strapped securely with a belt. Under these conditions, only the arms are actually involved in the throwing action. The ball is close to the chest with both hands, elbows flexed. (Figure 203).

Performance: Extend the elbows actively to throw the ball a maximum distance.

Scoring: The best of three trials is scored.

Other Suggested Medicine Ball Tests:
- forward, overhead throw
- between legs, forward throw
- between legs, backward throw

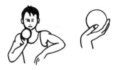

Figure 204.   Standing Shot Put

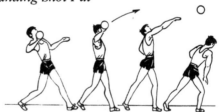

Figure 205.   Standing Shot Put

Equipment: 4 kg (9 lb.) for junior girls, 5 kg (12 lb.) for women and junior boys, and 7 kg (16 lb.) for senior male athletes.

Starting Postion (for right-hander): The athlete stands, left shoulder facing the direction of throw, left leg behind the throwing line (or edge of the circle), the shot held on the fingers, the shot resting on the shoulder against the neck and chin (Figure 204).

Performance: Put for maximum distance (Figure 205).

Scoring: Best of three trials.

Safety Factors: No athletes should be allowed in the throwing area.

148

Other Suggested Shot Throws (two arms):
- between legs, forward throw
- between legs, backward throw

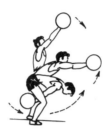

Figure 206. Heavy Bell Throws
Equipment: 5 kg (12 lb.) for junior girls, 10 kg (22 lb.) for women and
    junior boys, and 15 kg (33 lb.) for senior male athletes.
Starting Position: Two parallel benches, 50 cm (25 in) apart. The
    athlete stands with one foot on each bench, the bell being held by
    both hands, knees and hips slightly flexed (Figure 206).
    Performance: The bell is swung backwards, and then forwards,
    culminating with a throw at maximum distance.
Scoring: Best of three trials.

Note: Unless there are indoor bells available, this test must be
performed outdoors.
Safety Factors: No athletes should be allowed in the throwing area.

Leg Tests
Power Tests
    Standing Long Jump
Equipment: Sand pit, or gym floor (marked in centimetres up to 300
    cm), or in inches up to 125 in.).
Starting Position: Feet slightly apart, toes behind the jumping line.
Performance: Using arm action to assist, the performer jumps as far as
    possible (Figure 89).
Scoring: Record to the nearest inch (or cm) the distance from the
    jumping line to the heel mark in the best of 2 trials.

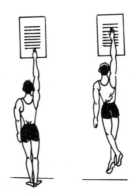

Figure 207.   Vertical Jump

Equipment and Marking: Vertical jump board 30 cm x 150 cm
    (1 ft x 5 ft) marked in centimetres (inches), mounted on a wall.

Starting Position: Subject stands flat-footed facing the wall and reaches
    as high as possible over his head. Mark this height and move to a
    comfortable position away from the wall with either side to the wall.

Performance: Subject jumps as high as possible and touches the board
    at the maximum height of the jump. The body should not be turned.

Scoring: Measurement is to the nearest centimetre (inch) from the
    standing height to the jump height marked on the board (Gledhill,
    1987).

Standing Triple Jump

Equipment: A sand pit or 12 m (25 ft) floor space.

Starting Postion: The subject stands with one foot firmly planted just
    behind the take-off line. The other foot and the rest of body may be
    in any position desired.

Performance: The subject, using the arms to assist, jumps as far forward
    as possible in a consecutive hop, step, and land.

Scoring: Measurement is in centimetres (feet and inches), to the nearest
    centimetre (inch), from the take-off line to the heel of the foot, or
    the portion of the body nearest to the take-off line.

Power - Endurance Tests
    Penta-Jumps (five jumps)
    Deca-jumps (ten jumps)

Note: Both the penta- and deca-jumps are performed in a triple-jump
manner, where the first is a hop, the last a jump (as in long jump), and
in between are a series of steps. It can be performed from standing or
with three or five running steps. The longer attempt of two is recorded.

150

Data Recording Sheet

Medicine Balls (MB) Throws   **Score:**

   1. MB chest throw   _____ ft

   2. MB forward, overhead throw   _____ ft

   3. MB between legs, forward throw   _____ ft

   4. MB between legs, backward throw   _____ ft

Shot Put

   1. Standing short put   _____ ft

   2. Between legs, forward throw   _____ ft

   3. Between legs, backward throw   _____ ft

Heavy Bell Throws

   1. Female (12/22 lbs)   _____ ft

   2. Male (22/33 lbs)   _____ ft

Standing Long Jump   _____ in.

Standing High Jump   _____ in.

Standing Triple Jump   _____ ft

Power-Endurance

   1. Penta-jumps   _____ ft

   2. Deca-jumps   _____ ft

Norms for Power Tests

1. Male College Physical Education Students (Gledhill, 1987)

%	Med-Ball Throw (ft)	St. Long Jump (ft)	Vertical Jump (ft)	Standing Triple Jump (ft)	Shot Put (ft)
100	48.2	9.5	3.0	28.0	47.0
95	23.0	8.8	2.4	26.0	37.6
90	22.0	8.6	2.3	25.3	36.0
85	21.0	8.5	2.1	24.9	35.0
80	20.3	8.4	2.1	24.5	34.0
75	19.0	8.3	2.0	24.0	33.2
70	18.0	8.2	2.0	24.0	33.0
65	17.0	8.1	2.0	23.5	32.5
60	16.0	8.0	1.9	23.0	32.0
55	16.0	8.0	1.9	22.8	31.5
50	15.0	7.9	1.8	22.5	31.0
45	14.9	7.8	1.8	22.0	30.0
40	14.3	7.7	1.8	21.9	29.7
35	14.0	7.5	1.8	21.2	29.0
30	13.9	7.4	1.7	21.0	32.0
25	13.0	7.2	1.7	20.5	27.5
20	13.0	7.1	1.7	20.0	26.7
15	12.4	7.0	1.7	20.0	26.0
10	11.9	7.0	1.5	19.0	25.0
5	10.8	6.6	1.4	18.0	24.0

Norms for Power Tests

2. Female College Physical Education Students (Gledhill, 1987)

%	Med-Ball Throw (ft)	St. Long Jump (ft)	Vertical Jump (ft)	Standing Triple Jump (ft)	Shot Put (ft)
100	42.0	9.5	3.2	27.5	30.4
95	31.0	7.3	2.0	20.1	27.0
90	29.2	7.1	1.7	19.8	25.1
85	27.8	6.9	1.6	19.6	24.1
80	26.3	6.8	1.6	19.1	23.7
75	25.5	6.6	1.5	18.8	23.0
70	25.0	6.6	1.5	18.4	23.0
65	24.0	6.5	1.4	18.1	22.0
60	23.0	6.5	1.4	18.0	21.6
55	22.5	6.4	1.4	17.7	21.0
50	22.0	6.3	1.4	17.2	21.0
45	21.2	6.2	1.3	17.1	21.0
40	21.0	6.1	1.3	17.0	20.0
35	20.0	6.0	1.3	17.0	20.0
30	19.0	6.0	1.3	16.6	19.2
25	19.0	5.9	1.2	16.0	19.0
20	18.5	5.9	1.2	16.0	18.0
15	18.0	5.6	1.1	15.4	17.2
10	17.0	5.5	1.0	15.0	17.0
5	10.8	5.3	0.9	14.2	15.0

Norms for Power Tests for Track and Field Athletes
Age 16 - 17
(Romanian Athletics Federation, 1986)

Events:

Sprinting	Male	Female
1. 30 m sprint (low start)	4.0 sec	4.4 sec
2. Standing long jump	2.70 m	2.30 m
3. Standing triple jump	8.00 m	6.70 m
4. Penta-jump	14.00 m	12.00 m
Long Jump		
1. 30 m sprint (low start)	4.2 sec	4.6 sec
2. Standing long jump	2.80 m	2.40 m
3. Standing triple jump	8.40 m	7.00 m
Long Jump		
1. 30 m sprint (flying start)	2.8 sec	3.3 sec
2. Standing vertical jump	.65 m	.50 m
3. Standing long jump	2.80 m	2.40 m
4. Standing triple jump	8.20 m	7.00 m
Triple Jump		
1. 30 m sprint (flying start)	2.90 sec	3.40 sec
2. Standing triple jump	8.60 m	7.30 m
Shot Put		
1. 30 m sprint (low start)	4.30 sec	4.70 sec
2. Standing long jump	2.65 m	2.30 m
3. Standing shot put	12.50 m	10.50 m

(12 lbs for male, 9 lbs for female athletes).

154

Norms for Power Tests for Track and Field
(USSR Olympic Athletes, 1988)

		Male				Female	
		H.J.	L.J.	T.J.	P.V.	H.J.	L.J.
S **P** **E** **E** **D**	30m flying start	—	2.7-2.8	—	—	—	3.0-3.2
	40m low start	4.7-4.8	—	4.5	4.6	5.4-5.5	—
	40 with the P.V.	—	—	—	4.9	—	—
P **O** **W** **E** **R**	Vertical jump Swing arms (cm)	—	—	—	85	—	—
	Penta jump (m) with 6-7 steps	22.00	23.00	24.50	22.10	18.50-19.00	18.80-19.30

Legend:

H.J.	=	high jump
L.J.	=	long jump
T.J.	=	triple jump
P.V.	=	pole vault

GLOSSARY OF TERMS

REFERENCES

INDEX

GLOSSARY OF TERMS

Amortization Phase
The amortization phase is the eccentric or yielding phase of an activity. Amortization occurs just prior to the active or push-off phase of an activity, and includes the time from ground contact to the reverse movement.

Concentric/Isotonic/Dynamic Contraction
A concentric/isotonic/dynamic contraction is a contraction in which the muscle develops tension while shortening.

Eccentric Contraction
An eccentric contraction is a contraction in which the muscle develops tension while lengthening.

Extrafusal Fibres
Commonly referred to as simply muscle fibre, they are called extrafusal fibres only to differentiate them from intrafusal fibres. These fibres develop external tension.

Intrafusal Fibres
Located within the muscle spindle, the intrafusal fibres have a contractile component which maintains the sensitivity of the muscle spindle at various lengths. Intrafusal fibres do not participate in developing external tension, but instead serve as a sensory organ.

Muscle Receptors
Muscle receptors are proprioceptors which monitor systems related specifically to skeletal muscles. These receptors include the Golgi tendon organ and muscle spindle, which send information to higher brain centres about muscle tension, static length, velocity of stretch, and pressure.

Muscle Spindle

One of the most elaborately structured intrinsic receptors of the body is the muscle spindle. It conveys information about the muscle to the CNS. It is located within the muscle in-parallel to the extrafusal fibres. This feature allows the muscle spindle to be sensitive to muscle length. The muscle spindle monitors the muscle's static length, change in length, and pressure.

Plyometrics

Plyometrics are drills or exercises aimed at linking sheer strength and speed of movement to produce an explosive-reactive type of movement. The term is often used to refer to jumping drills and depth jumping, but plyometrics can include any drill or exercise utilizing the stretch reflex to produce an explosive reaction.

Proprioceptor

Any mechanism which monitors change in the body is a proprioceptor. Proprioceptors conduct sensory reports to the CNS from muscles, tendons, ligaments, and joints. These sensory reports are about orientation, angle of joints, degree of muscle shortening/lengthening, and velocity of stretch.

Stretch or Myotatic Reflex

A stretch or myotatic reflex is a reflex which responds to the rate of muscle stretch. This reflex has the fastest-known response to a stimulus (in this case the rate of muscle stretch). The myotatic/stretch reflex elicits contraction of homonymous muscle and synergist muscles (those surrounding the stretched muscle which produce the same movement), and inhibition of the antagonist muscles.

REFERENCES

Asmussen, E. (1979). Muscle fatigue. *Medicine and Science in Sports*, **11**(4), 313-321.

Astrand, P.O. & Rodhal K. (1986). *Textbook of work physiology: Physiological bases of exercise* (3rd ed). New York: McGraw Hill, 756

Atha, J.(1981). Strengthening muscle. *Exercise and Sport Sciences Reviews* **9**, 1-73.

Berstrom, J., Hermansen, L., Hultman E., Saltin, B. (1967). Diet, muscle glycogen and physical performance. *Acta Physiologica Scandinavica*, **71**, 140-150.

Blattner, S.E. & Noble, L. (1979). Relative effects of isokinetic and plyometric training on vertical jumping performance. *Research Quarterly,* **50**(4), 583-588.

Bigland-Ritchie, B., Johnson, R., Lippold, C.J., Woods, J.J. (1983). Contractile speed and EMG changes during fatigue of sustained maximal voluntary contractions. *Journal of Neurophysiology*, **50**(1), 313-324.

Bompa, T.O. (1983). *Theory and methodology of training: the key to athletic performance.* Dubuque,Iowa: Kendall/Hunt Pub. Co., 280.

Bompa, T. (1988) *Myotatic stretch training as a power training method for track cycling.* Seoul, Korea: Olympic Scientific Congress, Sept 9-15.

Bosco, C., Komi, P.V., (1981). Influence of countermovement amplitude in potentiation of muscular performance. In: Morecki, A. et al. (eds), *Biomechanics VII: proceedings of the 7th Congress of Biomechanics*, Warsaw, Poland, Baltimore: University Park Press, 129-135.

Bosco, C., Luhtanen, P., Komi, P.V. (1976). Kinetics and kinematics of the take-off in the long jump, In P. Komi (Ed.) *Biomechanics V-B.* Baltimore, Md: University Park Press, 174-180.

Bosco, C. Komi, P.V., Ito, A. (1981). Prestretch potentiation of human skeletal muscle during ballistic movement. *Acta Physiologica Scandinavica*, **111**(2), 135-140.

Bosco, C., Viitasalo, J.T., Komi, P.V., Luhtanen, P. (1982) . Combined effect of elastic energy and myoelectrical potentiation during stretch-shortening cycle exercise. *Acta Physiologica Scandinavica,* **114**(4), Apr 1982, 557-565.

Bosco, C., Zanon, S., Rusko, H., Dal Monte, A. (1984). The influence of extra load on the mechanical behavior of skeletal muscle. *European Journal of Applied Physiology and Occupational Physiology, 53*(2), 149-154.

Brooks, G.A., Brauner, K. T., Cassens, R.G. (1973). Glycogen synthesis and metabolism of lactic acid after exercise. *American Journal of Physiology, 224*(5), 1162-1166.

Cavagna, G. (1970). Elastic bounce of the body. *Journal of Applied Physiology, 29*(3), 279-282.

Cavagna, G., Disman, B., Margaria, R. (1968). Positive work done by a previously stretched muscle. *Journal of Applied Physiology, 24*(1), 21-32.

Chu, D. (1984). Plyometric exercise. *National Strength & Conditioning Association Journal, 5*(6), 56-59; 61-63.

Chu, D. (1983). Plyometrics: the link between strength and speed. *National Strength & Conditioning Association Journal, 5*(2), 20-21.

Clutch, D., Wilton, M., McGown, C., Bryce, T. (1983). Effect of depth jumps and weight training on leg strength and vertical jump. *Research Quarterly for Exercise & Sport, 54*(1), 5-10.

Gledhill, N. (1987). *Fitness Assessment.* Toronto, Ont.: York University Press.

Gollhofer, A., Komi, P.V., Miyashita, M., Aura, O. (1987). Fatigue during stretch-shortening cycle exercises: changes in mechanical performance of human skeletal muscle. *International Journal of Sports Medicine, 8*(2), 71-78.

Gollhofer, A., Fujitsuka, P.A., Miyashita, M. (1987). Fatigue during stretch-shortening II. Changes in neuromuscular activation patterns of human skeletal muscle. *International Journal of Sports Medicine, 8*(suppl 1), 38-47.

Haeekkinen, K. & Komi, P.V. (1983). Alterations of mechanical characteristics of human skeletal muscle during strength training. *European Journal of Applied Physiology and Occupational Physiology, 50*(2), 161-172.

Harre, D. (ed) (1982). *Traininglehre. (Principles of sports training: introduction to the theory and methods of training)* (1st ed). Berlin: Sportverlag, 231.

Karlson, J., & Saltin, B. (1971). Diet, muscle glycogen and endurance performance. *Journal of Applied Physiology,* **31**(2), 203-206.

Katschajov, G. (1976). Rebound Jumps. *Modern Athlete and Coach.* July.

Komi, P.V. and Burskirk, E.R. (1972). Effect of eccentric and concentric muscle conditioning on tension and electrical activity of human muscle. *Ergonomics,* **15**(4), 417-434.

Lindh, M. (1979). Increase of muscle strength from isometric quadriceps exercises at different knee angles. *Scandinavian Journal of Rehabilitative Medicine,* **11**(1), 33-36.

Mathews, D.K. & Fox, E.L. (1976). *Physiological basis of physical education and athletics.* Philadelphia: W.B. Sanders, 577.

Matsuda, J.J., Zernicke, R.F., Vailus, A.C. Pedrini, V.A., Pedrini-Mille, A. Maynard, J.A. (1986). Structural and mechanical adaptation of immature bone to strenuous exercise. *Journal of Applied Physiology,* **60**(6), 2028-2034.

O'Connell, A.L. & Gardner, E.B. (1972). *Understanding the scientific basis of human movement.* Baltimore: William & Wilkins, 264.

Ozolin, N.G., (1971). Athlete's training system for competition. *Phyzkultura i Sport.:* Moscow.

Pollock, M.L. (1973). Quantification of endurance training programs, In: *Exercise and Sport Sciences Review* **1**, 155-188.

Powers, S.K., Dodd, S. Beadle, R.E. (1985). Oxygen uptake kinetics in trained athletes differing in VO2 max. *European Journal of Applied Physiology and Occupational Physiology,* **54**(3), 306-308.

Radcliffe, J.C. & Farentinos, R.C. (1985). *Plyometrics: explosive power training* (2nd ed). Champaign, Ill.: Human Kinetics Publishers, 127.

Schmidtbleicher, D. & Gollhofer, A. (1982). Neuromuskulaere Untersuchungen zur bestimmung individueller belastungsgroessen fuer ein tiefsprungtraining (Neuromuscular examination of the determination of individual training loads for jump training). *Leistungssport,* **12**(4), 298-307.

Schmidtbleicher, D. (1980). *Maximalkraft und bewegungsschelligkeit*. Bad Homburg: Limpert Verlag.

Schmidtbleicher, D. (1984). Sportliches Krafttraining *Jung, Haltung und Bewengung bei Menschen*:: Berlin.

Schroder, W. (1978). Summary of strength and power development. *Modern Athlete and Coach*, **16**(4), 9-10.

Setchenov, I.M. (1935). *On the question of the increase of the human muscle working capacity*. Selected works: Moscow.

Tschiene, P. (1980). Modern trends in strength training, In: Jarver, J., *Throws*, Los Altos, CA: Tafnews Press, 17-19.

Verkoshansky, V. (1967). Are depth jumps useful?. *Track and Field*, **12**, 9.

Verkoshansky, V. (1969). Perspectives in the improvement of speed-strength preparation of jumpers. *Review of Soviet Education and Sports*, **4**(2), 28-29.

Verkhoshansky, V. & Tatyan, V. (1983). Speed-strength preparationof future champions. *Soviet sports review*, **18**(4), 166-170.

Wilt, F. (1978). Plyometrics: what is is and how it works. *Modern Athlete and Coach*, **16**(2), 9-12.

Yakovlev, N.N. (1967). *Sports Biochemistry*, Leipzig: DHFK.

Young, W.; Marino, W. (1985). The importance of bounding in the jumping events. *Modern Athlete and Coach*, **23**(2), 11-13.

Zanon, S. (1977). Consideration for determining some parametric values of the relations between maximum isometric relative strength and elastic realtive strength for planning and controlling the long jumper's conditioning training, *Athletic Coach*, **11**(4), 14-20.

APPENDIX   1

CHARTS FOR DETERMINING THE STARTING
POINT IN PLYOMETRIC TRAINING
(made by Yus Omar, 1994)

The values suggested by the following charts can be used by the coach/ athlete to deterning entry level/starting sets/reps/loads for the various plyometric exercises mentioned. It is recommended that the coach/athlete follow a careful progression from the determined starting point. If this is not the case then injury may ensue.

The progression of sets and reps provides the coach/athlete with a guideline to ensure that the progression is not too demanding/easy.

Physical maturity must be determined, as well as strength training background, when dealing with all athletes, especially those that are pre-pubescent, pubescent, post-pubescent, or older.

As stated in the titles of each chart, these values are ''suggested'', and therefore care, intelligence, experience should be exercised when implementing any of the plyometric exercises and their corresponding starting values.

Please do not jump ahead or skip any progression as outlined in this book. By overlooking such information the athlete may be putting him/ herself at risk of physical injury.

BENCH X BODY WEIGHT	PLYOMETRIC EXERCISE	STARTING SETS REPS	SETS /WK	REPS /WK
$1/_4 - 1/_2$	-	-	-	-
$1/_2 - 3/_4$	-	-	-	-
$3/_4 - 1$	CLAPPING PUSH UP**	2-3	2-3	-
$1 - 1^1/_4$	$1/_2$ PLYO PUSH UP	2-3(4)	2-3	-
$1^1/_4 - 1^1/_2$	"	3-4	2-3(4)	-
$1^1/_2 - 1^3/_4$	(R)	4-5	3-4	-
$1^3/_4 - 2$	"	4-5	3-4(5)	-
$2 - 2^1/_4$	"	5-6	4-5	-
$2^1/_4 - 2^1/_2$	"	5-6	4-5(6)	-
$2^1/_2 - 2^3/_4$	"	6-7	5-6	-
$2^3/_4 - 3$	"	6-7	5-6	-
$3 - 3^1/_4$	"	7-8	6-7(8)	-

R=REACTIVE (DECREASE SETS BY AT LEAST 1-2(3))

BENCH X BODY WEIGHT	PLYOMETRIC EXERCISE	STARTING SETS REPS	SETS /WK	REPS /WK

CLAPPING PUSH UP

BENCH X BODY WEIGHT	PLYOMETRIC EXERCISE	STARTING SETS REPS	SETS /WK	REPS /WK
$^3/_4$ - 1	CLAPPING PUSH UP		2-3	2-3
1 - $1^1/_4$	-		2-3(4)	2-3(4)
$1^1/_4$ - $1^1/_2$	-		4-5	3-4
$1^1/_2$ - $1^3/_4$	-		5-6	3-4(5)
$1^3/_4$ - 2	-		6-7	4-5
2 - $2^1/_4$	-		6-7	5-6
$2^1/_4$ - $2^1/_2$	-		7-8	5-6(7)
$2^1/_2$ - $2^3/_4$	-		7-8	7-8
$2^3/_4$ - 3	-		7-8(9)	7-8(9)
3 - $3^1/_4$	-		8-9	8-9

FULL PLYO PUSH UP

BENCH X BODY WEIGHT	PLYOMETRIC EXERCISE	STARTING SETS REPS	SETS /WK	REPS /WK
$1^3/_4$ - 2	FULL PLYO PUSH UP		2-3	2-3
2 - $2^1/_4$	"		2-3(4)	2-3(4)
$2^1/_4$ - $2^1/_2$	(R)		4-5	3-4
$2^1/_2$ - $2^3/_4$	"		4-5	3-4(5)
$2^3/_4$ - 3	"		5-6	4-5
3 - $3^1/_4$	"		5-6	4-5(6)

R=REACTIVE FULL PLYO PUSH UP (DECREASE SETS BY AT LEAST 1-2(3))

NOTE: The Number of reps done per session and per week increase depending upon technique and contact time during execution.

The increase in sets will depend upon age, caliber of athlete and prior plyometric training experience.

PLYO INTENSITY	PARALLEL SQUAT X BODY WT.	STARTING* SETS REPS**	%REPS /WK***	%SETS /WK
5	$\frac{1}{4}$	1-2	-	-
5	$\frac{1}{4}$ - $\frac{1}{2}$	2-3	-	-
5	$\frac{1}{2}$ - $\frac{3}{4}$	(2)3-4	-	-
5	$\frac{3}{4}$ - 1	(3)4-5	-	5
5	1 - $1\frac{1}{4}$	(4)5-6	-	5-10
5/4	$1\frac{1}{4}$ - $1\frac{1}{2}$	(2)3-4	-	10-15
5/4	$1\frac{1}{2}$ - $1\frac{3}{4}$	(2)3-4	-	15-20
5/4	$1\frac{3}{4}$ - 2	(3)4-5	-	15-20
5/4	2 - $2\frac{1}{4}$	(3)4-5	-	20-25
3/4	$2\frac{1}{4}$ - $2\frac{1}{2}$	2-3	-	10-15
3/4	$2\frac{1}{2}$ - $2\frac{3}{4}$	(2)3-4	-	(15)20-25
2/3	$2\frac{3}{4}$ - 3	(2)3-4	-	10-15 (20)
2/3	3 - $3\frac{1}{4}$	(3)4-5	-	20-25 (30)
2/3	$3\frac{1}{4}$ - $3\frac{1}{2}$	(4)5-6	-	30-35 (40)
1/2	$3\frac{1}{2}$ - $3\frac{3}{4}$	(2)3-4	-	30-35 (40)
1/2	$3\frac{3}{4}$ - 4	(2)3-4	-	30-35(40)
1/2	4 - $4\frac{1}{4}$	(3)4-5	-	30-35 (40)
1/2	$4\frac{1}{4}$ - $4\frac{1}{2}$	(3)4-5	-	30-35 (40)
1/2	$4\frac{1}{2}$ - $4\frac{3}{4}$	(4)5-6	-	30-35 (40)

NOTE ** PER SESSION
***Reps will be determined by technique and contact time during execution of the plyometric exercise.

M	T	W	T	F	SA	SU
		2				
1				3		

1)INTRODUCE PLYO. EX. (**TIMES1/2)
2)INCREASE PLYO. EX. (**)
3)ADAPTATION TO PLYO EX. (*TIMES 1/2-1/4)

PLYOMETRIC HEIGHT INCREASE BASED UPON THE 5 PLYOMETRIC INTENSITIES

PLYO. INTENSITY	PARALLEL SQUAT X BODY WT.	HEIGHT INCREASE
5	$1 - 1\frac{1}{4}$	5CM/MONTH
5	$1\frac{1}{4} - 1\frac{1}{2}$	5CM/3WEEKS
5	$1\frac{1}{2} - 1\frac{3}{4}$	5CM/2WEEKS
5	$1\frac{3}{4} - 2$	5CM/WEEK
4	$2 - 2\frac{1}{4}$	5-10CM/MONTH
4	$2\frac{1}{4} - 2\frac{1}{2}$	5-10CM/3WEEK
4	$2\frac{1}{2} - 2\frac{3}{4}$	5-10/2 WEEK
4	$2\frac{3}{4} - 3$	5-10CM/WEEK
3(2 LEGS)	$2\frac{1}{4} - 2\frac{1}{2}$	5CM/MONTH
3(2 LEGS)	$2\frac{1}{2} - 2\frac{3}{4}$	5CM/3WEEKS
3(2 LEGS)	$2\frac{3}{4} - 3$	5CM/2WEEKS
3(2 LEGS)	$3 - 3\frac{1}{4}$	5CM/WEEK
3(1 LEG)	$2\frac{1}{2} - 2\frac{3}{4}$	5CM/MONTH
3(1 LEG)	$2\frac{3}{4} - 3$	5CM/3WEEKS
3(1 LEG)	$3 - 3\frac{1}{4}$	5CM/2 WEEKS
3(1 LEG)	$3\frac{1}{4} - 3\frac{1}{2}$	5CM/WEEK
2	$2\frac{1}{2} - 2\frac{3}{4}$	5-10CM/MONTH
2	$2\frac{3}{4} - 3$	5-10CM/3WEEK
2	$3 - 3\frac{1}{4}$	5-10CM/2 WEEK
2	$3\frac{1}{4} - 3\frac{1}{2}$	5-10CM/WEEK
1	$3 - 3\frac{1}{4}$	5-10CM/MONTH
1	$3\frac{1}{4} - 3\frac{1}{2}$	5-10CM/3 WEEK
1	$3\frac{1}{2} - 3\frac{3}{4}$	5-10CM/2 WEEK
1	$3\frac{3}{4} - 4$	5-10CM/WEEK

NOTE: Increase will also depend upon age, caliber of athlete and prior plyometric training background.

INDEX

A
Acceleration: 11, 12
Adaptation: 5, 6, 26, 27, 28, 29, 31, 32, 35, 36, 37, 38, 39, 45, 55, 63, 67, 74, 122
Aerobic energy system: 15, 16
Agonistic muscles: 19
Amortization phase: 10, 11, 12
Anaerobic alactic: 14, 15, 16, 32, 59
Anaerobic lactic: 15, 16, 32
Annual plan: 5, 43, 54, 55, 61, 64, 76
Antagonistic muscles: 19
B
Ballistic: 3, 12, 124
Baseball: 4, 64, 71, 75, 134, 145
Basketball: 4, 64, 74
Biological age: 34
Bounding exercises: 12, 42, 44, 47, 51, 75, 78, 79, 83, 87, 90, 98, 104
C
Carbohydrates: 15, 61
Centre of gravity: 1, 8,10,11,12
Chronological age: 34
Compensation: 28, 29, 30, 31
Concentric: 1, 4, 5, 6, 10, 11, 17, 18, 26, 104
Cross-training: 33
Crossed extensor reflex: 19
Contact phase: 6, 7
D
Depth jump: 6, 25, 45, 103
Drop (shock) jumps: 33, 42, 43, 44, 47, 64, 75, 77, 103, 114
E
Eccentric: 1, 5, 11, 17, 18, 19, 26, 104
Eccentric contraction: 4, 6
Endurance training: 15,16
Energy Systems: 1, 14, 16, 32, 33, 59, 62

F

Fast Twitch muscle fibre: 17, 33

Fatigue: 15, 16, 17, 26, 29, 31, 38, 47, 48, 53, 57, 58, 59, 61, 70, 142

Figure skating: 4, 52, 69, 71

Football: 4

Force-time curve: 7, 8

G

Glycogen: 15, 29, 59

Golf: 1, 4

Golgi tendon organ: 6, 18, 21, 23, 25

Gymnastics: 2, 7, 52, 69, 71, 74

H

High impact plyometrics (exercises): 42, 43, 44, 45, 64, 67, 68

High Jump: 4, 7, 11

Hypertrophy: 15, 28

I

Individualization: 33, 34, 35

Injury: 3, 5, 12, 13, 18, 27, 35, 40, 41, 44, 48, 50, 61, 76, 77, 119

Innervation: 5

Intensity: 5, 27, 29, 30, 31, 34, 39, 40, 42, 43, 44, 45, 48, 50, 54, 55, 56, 57, 59, 64, 67, 68, 72, 73, 74

Intensity of stimuli: 5, 28, 29, 39

Involution: 29, 36

Isokinetic: 17

Isometric: 17, 19, 33

Isotonic: 17

K

Kinetic energy: 6, 103

L

Lactic acid: 15, 29, 47, 48, 59

Load: 5, 34, 35, 36, 38, 39, 47, 55, 62, 63, 67

Long jump: 10, 11, 12, 43, 45, 97, 150

Low impact plyometrics (exercises): 43, 44, 46, 47, 64, 66, 68, 94

M

Macrocycle: 38

Medicine ball (throw): 43, 63, 67, 75, 121, 125, 126-134, 142-145, 147-149

Menstrual cycle: 35

Microcycle: 38, 54, 55, 56, 57, 58, 62
Motor neurons: 8
Motor units: 5, 6, 20, 26, 28
Multiple-response drills (MR): 47, 79
Muscle fibre: 5, 6, 19, 20, 21, 22, 23, 24, 26, 28, 33
Muscle fibre type: 17, 18, 19
Muscle spindle: 6, 20, 22, 23, 24, 25
Myotatic reflex: 6, 24, 26
Myotatic stretch reflex: 1, 6
N
Nervous impulse: 23, 24, 48, 52
Nervous system: 5, 20, 23, 26, 36, 52
Nervous system training: 47, 52
Neural stimulus/reflex/activation: 18, 19, 68
Neuro-muscular system: 3, 18, 27, 28, 36, 41, 42, 62
Neuro-muscular units: 7, 24, 42
O
Overcompensation: 28, 29, 30, 31, 57, 58, 59, 60, 68
Overload: 15, 37, 42
P
Peak force: 8, 12, 61
Peaking: 61, 64, 65, 68
Periodization: 1, 5, 13, 49, 61, 62, 63, 64, 66, 67, 70, 74
Power training: 3, 5, 9, 36, 45, 47, 59
Prime movers: 32, 33, 67
R
Reaction time/exercise: 5, 52, 53
Reactive jump: 7, 8, 36, 40, 42, 43, 44, 45, 47, 48, 64, 78, 103, 104, 105, 106, 108
Reactive power: 1, 41
Reactive training: 1, 3, 26, 55, 59, 66
Recovery: 26, 30, 35, 54, 59, 62
Reflex contraction: 19
Regeneration: 28, 37, 55, 62
Rest interval: 44, 47, 48
S
Sheringtonian neurophysiology: 19
Shock absorbing: 9, 10, 12, 40, 45, 125
"Shock" tension (machine): 43, 44, 47, 75, 77, 114, 116, 117, 118, 122, 124, 125, 139

Single-response drills (SR): 47, 79
Ski jumping/skiing: 4, 64, 71
Slow twitch muscle fiber: 17
Soccer: 64
Specificity: 32, 33, 70, 72, 73
Speed training: 15, 35, 45, 52, 53, 59
Squat jump: 7, 8
Step-type method: 37
Strength training: 8, 9, 12, 15, 19, 28, 33, 41, 45, 47, 54
Stretch reflex: 6, 10, 18, 24, 25
Stretching-shortening cycle: 1, 4, 5, 7, 8, 53, 64, 78
Swimming: 69, 71
T
Team Sports: 4, 71
Test; testing: 35, 38, 147-151
Throwing events: 4
Track and field: 2, 74
Tracking stimulus: 2, 5, 37
Triple jump: 12, 43, 72, 74, 84, 151
U
Unloading: 37, 38, 68
V
Volleyball: 4, 64
Volume (of training): 27, 34, 39, 52, 70, 72, 73
W
Weight training: 4, 6, 7, 8, 12
Wrestling/wrestler: 52, 74